If Not Now, When?

Reduce Weight

Create a Healthy Lifestyle in 90 Days

David Medansky

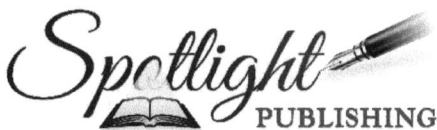

Spotlight PUBLISHING

Goodyear, Arizona

Medansky, David
If Not Now, When?
Reduce Weight
Create a Healthy Lifestyle in 90 Days

LCCN: 2019908434
Print ISBN: 978-1-7337388-5-9
Ebook ISBN: 978-1-7337388-6-6

Cover design: Suzette Vaughn

Copyediting: Penny Hill

Proofreading: Patrick Hodges
Interior design: Cindy Readnower

Published by MBK Enterprises, LLC | Spotlight Publishing

www.CreateYourThinnerSelf.com

If Not Now, When?

Reduce Weight - Create a Healthy a Lifestyle in 90 Days

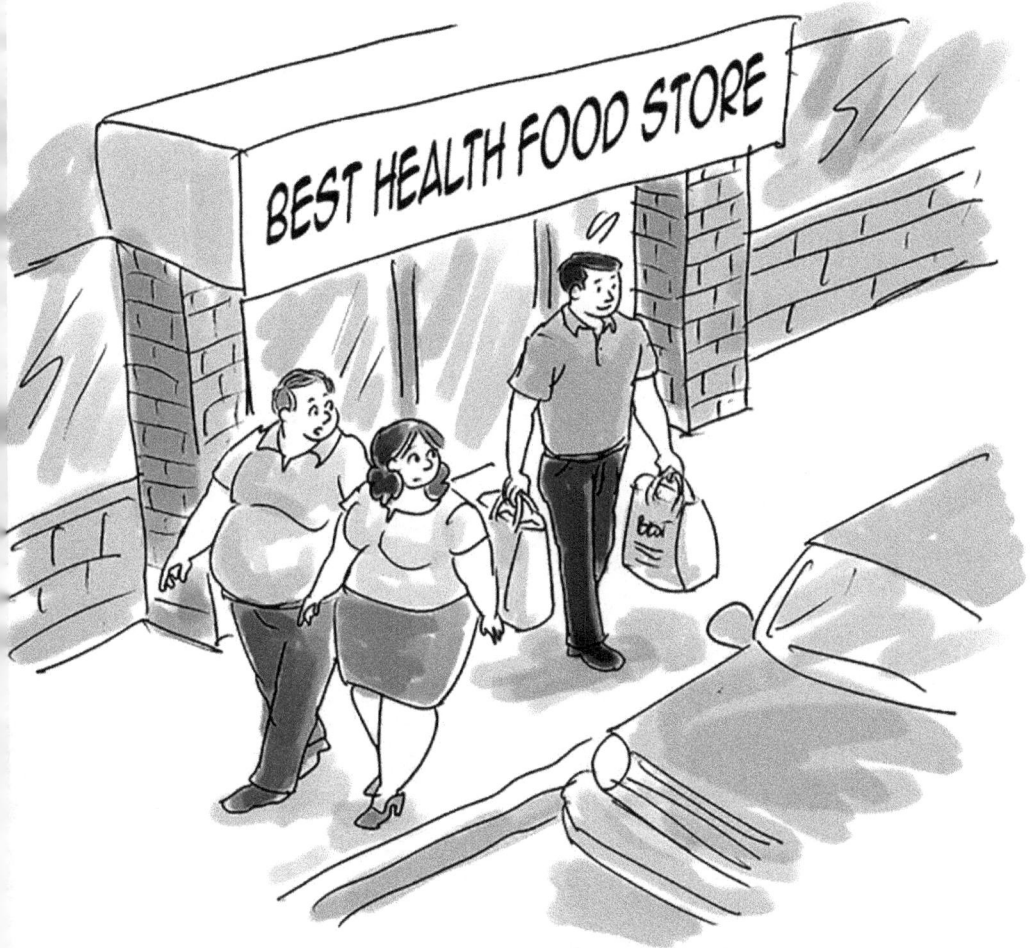

"POOR SCHMUCK, BOUGHT THAT HEALTH FOOD THING
HOOK, LINE, AND SINKER."

If we put off until tomorrow what we can do today, and tomorrow never comes, that means we will never do what needs to be done.

Top 10 Excuses Used to Delay Reducing Weight

1. I'll start after our vacation.
2. I'll start after the holidays.
3. Now's not the right time for me.
4. I'm too busy.
5. I'll start on Monday.
6. It's too expensive or healthy food cost too much.
7. I'll start after our company picnic or party.
8. I don't have time to follow a regimen.
9. Many people who lose weight gain it all back so why bother?
10. I'm always hungry and cranky on a diet.

"You must unlearn what you have learned." Yoda, Jedi Master

Only positive thoughts beyond this point.
Change is a choice

For my wife, Debra,
and my two daughters,
Michelle and Nikiana

Disclaimer

Before you implement any weight-reduction program or use any dietary, exercise, or health advice from this book, please consult a medical practitioner or qualified health professional.

All information provided in this book is intended for educational purposes only. Any health or dietary advice is *not* intended as a medical diagnosis or treatment. Statements contained in this book have not been evaluated by the Food and Drug Administration.

The author, publisher, and any other person involved in producing this book disclaim all liability and loss in conjunction with the content provided herein, as well as any and all liability for any products or services mentioned or recommended in this book. The information contained herein is subject to personal research and has been recorded as accurately as possible at the time of publication. Due to possible changes and availability of information provided to the public, you should not take any of the content as a source of reference without further research. The publisher and author are not responsible for any adverse effects or consequences resulting from the use of the suggestions, preparations, or procedures discussed in this book.

If you think you're suffering from any medical condition, then you should seek immediate medical attention.

Results may vary. Causes of being overweight or obese vary from person to person. No individual results should be deemed as typical.

The information contained in this book is based upon the research and personal experience of the author. It is not intended as a substitute for consulting with your physician or other healthcare provider. Any attempt to diagnose and treat an illness should be done under the direction of a healthcare professional.

WARNING: Losing weight using a low calorie or restricted diet can cause crankiness and irritability.

Table of Contents

Foreword by Lori Shemek, Ph.D.

Congratulations on taking action with your weight and health. Of all the self-empowering books you have available to choose from, you've chosen this one. What you are holding in your hand is not just another diet book; it is a true pathway to weight loss and health. Good for you for being proactive and seeking out the expert direction with author David Medansky.

Life is challenging and so is weight loss. The massive pool in this genre of books on the market is proof that people are searching for ways to lose weight in a way that works for them.

It's no surprise that the world's waistline is expanding and there are multiple reasons for this. The United States is considered the most obese developed country. Americans spend over $66 billion on weight loss products, yet 71 percent of the country is overweight and obese. This is a staggering statistic, but David has the answers because it isn't just one thing – there are multiple reasons and you will find the solutions.

When David Medansky asked me to write the foreword to his book *If Not Now, When?* I was honored and eager to share my message about his work, as he has been a significant part of changing the world's weight mindset in a healthy manner. I think of David as a true innovator and crusader for people's health.

He and I both know the weight woes that face the world right now. In fact, David was at one time very overweight and heading for a heart attack. He, like so many, struggled with multiple diets and in his mind 'failed' not realizing that he was utilizing the wrong fat loss information and essentially giving up with every 'failed' diet. How many of us can relate to that?

Not only does David personally know how challenging it can be to carry excess weight, but he also shares other's stories so poignantly in his book. He has put his expertise to work to change the conversation we are having about weight gain and what has been proven to solve it. Additionally, David makes it clear that whatever weight and health challenges you are experiencing, you are not alone and there *is* a solution.

For decades I've assisted clients who have struggled with their weight. My journey has found me on national television, in print media, on the radio or with my own-authored books, lending my expertise to the serious conversation of weight gain and inflammation that affects so many lives. I have found that in the majority of cases, people often know what to do, but they really struggle with the discipline part of shedding weight or they are missing pieces of the weight loss puzzle. So what happens? They fall for quick fixes, fad diets that are low-calorie, yo-yo dieting, diet pills, over-hyped exercise programs, expensive gym memberships, and fat loss procedures. This is where David's book stands widely apart from the rest. He wants you to create a *lifestyle* not a series of excuses. He separates the myths from the facts to take you to success.

Why lose weight? We all know that being overweight is not a punishable offense or lowers your value as a person. However, carrying excess weight can affect very important aspects of your day-to-day living such as your health, your ability to do and even enjoy activities. Your self-esteem and confidence level can be eroded and in fact, excess weight can impact most every area of your life.

I know that when you say you want to lose weight, what you really mean is that you want to be able to play with your children or walk up the stairs without losing your breath, you want to look in the mirror and feel good about that person staring back at you, you want to be able to sit in an airline seat comfortably, you also want to live a healthier, stronger and longer life. You want, in the end, to live a quality life.

David Medansky asks us this question "If not now, when?" We all have excuses that can stop us in our tracks, but we must answer his question. Are we going to continue replaying the same choices leading to the same outcome? Albert Einstein once said, "The definition of insanity is repeating the same behaviors and expecting a different outcome."

Stop the madness and recognize that when you have expert, well-researched quality information, you take action and you allow David's wisdom to guide you, the excess fat you are carrying will finally be a thing of the past.

Know that from this day forward, each one of us has the ability to take control of our eating, our choices and ultimately create a life we love.

Lori Shemek, Ph.D., CNC
Bestselling author of Fire-Up Your Fat Burn! and How to Fight FATflammation!

Chapter 1

Tomorrow Never Comes

It is better to offer no excuse than a bad one.
George Washington

In the movie *Rocky II*, Rocky Balboa's wife, Adrian (Talia Shire), wakes up from a coma and tells Rocky (Sylvester Stallone), "Win." Upon hearing Adrian tell Rocky to "Win," Rocky's manager, Mickey, (Burgess Meredith), says, "What are we waiting for?" The question posed to you if you're wanting or needing to lose weight is, "What are you waiting for?" Because if you're not going to start now, when will you start?

The biggest regret people have about losing weight is not starting a year earlier.

The second biggest regret about attaining a healthy weight is not starting now.

With respect to weight reduction, there are three types of people: 1) those who think about losing weight but do nothing, 2) those who talk endlessly about losing weight but do nothing, and 3) those who act to reduce weight. Which one are you?

Darren Hardy, New York Times best-selling author of *The Compound Effect* and renowned success mentor, in an episode of his *Darren Daily* podcast, asks a poignant question, "What will happen if I do this for 30 days? Will I be glad I did or regret I didn't?" The question I'll ask you is, if you start to apply the principles provided in this book for 30 days – or ideally 90 days -- will you be glad you did, or regret you didn't?

There is never a perfect or right time to begin shedding your unwanted and unhealthy weight because tomorrow never comes. Have you used the excuse to justify delaying your weight loss journey saying, "I'll start on Monday?" Or, "I'll start after the holidays?" "After our vacation?" You get the idea.

Ask yourself this, "If I delay and put off until tomorrow what I can start today, what might happen?" Here's a hint to your answer. Tomorrow never comes until it's too late. It means if you keep putting off until tomorrow what you can start today and if tomorrow never comes, you'll never start.

Have you promised yourself you'd lose weight? Probably, because most people make a New Year's resolution to diet. Studies and surveys that were done in recent years show the most common aspirations for a new year in the U.S. are to lose weight, eat healthier, get more exercise, quit smoking, and save more money.

Did you keep your promise?

It's a tough one to keep. I know. I've been there.

If you did lose weight, have you kept it off? I'm guessing probably not since almost 90 percent of people who start a diet, whether it be at New Year's or another time, quit after a few days. Some after a few months.

In this book, you will learn the importance of reducing weight and *what* to do to achieve a healthy weight. But, more importantly, *how* to do it and how to maintain it once you succeed. We'll delve into the mental, emotional and psychological aspects of weight loss.

I realize the information presented here might not be for everyone. But you may know someone, perhaps a friend, colleague, aunt, uncle, niece or nephew who can benefit from this information. If you do, please share this information with them.

I Did It. So Can You

Hello, my name is David Medansky. If you look at me now, you'd never suspect I was fat. But, at one time, I was.

Maybe some of you were like me. That being, we were fit and trim when we were younger. But, as with many of us, life got in the way. Some of you, like myself, may have gotten lazy or self-indulgent. Maybe you're like me and stopped exercising. Or started eating more junk food and fast foods because it's more convenient. Without realizing it, your weight crept up on you, just like it happened to me.

Like many of you, I struggled with weight issues and dieting. I tried and tried, but no matter what I did or what diet I attempted, I failed.

If I did lose weight, I couldn't keep it off. Instead of eating one scoop of ice cream, I'd eat an entire pint in one sitting. Or, I'd consume an entire canister of Pringles. I was disgusted with myself. I couldn't believe my pants size ballooned up. But then, something happened to turn my life around.

In July 2016, my doctor told me, based on my lab results, I had a 95 percent chance of having a heart attack. He gave me two choices: 1) either lose weight or 2) find a new doctor because he didn't want me dying on his shift.

In most things, I'm pleased to be in the 95th percentile – but not if it meant I was likely to die. Suddenly, my being 217 pounds was more than just embarrassing, it was lethal.

With that sword hanging over my head, I made the decision to shed my unwanted and unhealthy pounds. That began my weight-reduction journey. During the next four months, I lost 50 pounds and reduced my body weight by more than 25 percent. Now, I feel great and have more energy.

Would you like to feel better or have more energy?

I believe it's my duty and obligation to help others attain a healthy weight, so they don't worry and suffer like I used to or be at risk like I was. I've made it my mission to help others reduce weight in a healthy and sustainable manner.

Woody Allen is credited with saying, "Eighty percent of success in life is just showing up." Thank you for showing up and reading this book.

What Diets Cost You

Americans spend more than $66 billion each year on weight-loss products and programs, purchasing everything from diet pills to meal plans to swanky gym memberships. Yet, according to the U.S. Center for Disease Control and Prevention (CDC), 155 million Americans are overweight. Loosely translated, that's more than 71 percent of American adults of whom 41 percent are clinically obese. And it's getting worse.

What this means for you is if you're at a social gathering with ten other people, seven of you are overweight and four of you are clinically obese. Look around you and observe other people. What do you see? If you're honest with yourself, you'll observe more overweight people than at any other time in history. Think about that for a minute. Seven out of every ten U.S. adults are overweight. And, that does not include kids.

Over 43 million Americans start a diet or weight-loss program each year. However, 90 to 95 percent of diets fail. People tend to blame themselves rather than the diet.

Can you relate to that?

W. Edward Deming, known for systems, processes, and improvement to products and services said, "85 percent of the reasons for failure are deficiencies in the system and process rather than the employee."

Deming also said, "It is not enough to do your best; you must know what to do, and then do your best." And, "If you can't describe what you are doing as a process, you don't know what you're doing."

Being Overweight in America Is an Epidemic

Now is the time to improve your eating behaviors, habits and lifestyle because being overweight in America is an epidemic. We no longer have a health care crisis. It's more like disease care. Making the decision to reduce weight can change your life for the better and improve your overall health. Taking measures to achieve a healthy weight and maintain it is a choice.

If you choose not to make the effort to reduce weight you put yourself at a higher risk for chronic disease and illnesses such as:

- Type 2 diabetes
- High blood pressure
- Heart attack
- Stroke
- Certain types of cancer
- Liver failure
- Sleep apnea

- Osteoarthritis, among other ailments.

A study presented at the Society of General Internal Medicine 2017 Annual Meeting found that obesity has caused up to 47 percent more life-years lost than tobacco. The lead author of the study, Glen Taksler, Ph.D. looked into the underlying cause of a patient's death to understand the contributing factors. Dr. Taksler said, "The reality is, while we may know the proximate cause of a patient's death, for example, breast cancer or heart attack, we don't always know the contributing factor(s), such as tobacco use, obesity, alcohol and family history." The study examined each major cause of death. They identified a root cause to understand whether there was a way a person could have lived longer. The conclusion being overweight now causes more deaths than smoking.

Think about that. Obesity now causes more deaths than smoking. And, seven out of every ten U.S. adult are overweight and four of those ten, are clinically obese. Sobering statistics.

Researchers found that one in five deaths worldwide is linked to unhealthy eating habits. What you eat, and don't eat, may pose a bigger threat to your health than smoking, drinking, and other common risk factors for premature death. An extensive new study on diet trends around the globe ties poor eating habits to 11 million deaths around the world in 2017. The research, published in April 2019 in the journal, *The Lancet*, reported that bad eating habits were the primary factor that contributed to deaths linked to heart disease, Type 2 diabetes, and cancer.

Seventy percent of Americans (seven out of every ten) who are in the hospital are there because of their dietary habits and lifestyles. The sad part, much of it is preventable.

A 2009 study published in *The American Journal of Medicine* found that almost two-thirds of bankruptcies in the United States had a medical cause.

If you think it's expensive to eat healthy, you'd be wrong. Think of the costs of poor eating habits. It's expensive to get sick. The average out-of-pocket cost (after the insurance pays) per hospital stay after a heart attack is about $20,000.

Z

Why wait until you get a disease or medical condition that puts you in the hospital when you can significantly reduce the risk and possibly prevent it simply by reducing weight? And, if you shed those unwanted and extra pounds, you'll feel better, have more energy, and probably want to be more active.

Here's another sobering fact – 80 percent (that's 8 out of 10) men and women over age 50 are pre-diabetic or diabetic. Diabetes is the 6th leading cause of death for men and women. Over a third of people with diabetes do not know they have it. That's why diabetes is sometimes referred to as the "silent killer." Being overweight is the number one factor in increasing your risk of developing Type 2 diabetes. Type 2 diabetes is often a lifestyle disease, and it's preventable.

According to the Center for Disease Control and Prevention, "A person with diabetes is at high risk of heart disease, stroke, and other serious complications, such as kidney failure, blindness, and amputation of a toe, foot, or leg. In the last 20 years, the number of adults diagnosed with diabetes has more than tripled as the U.S. population has aged and become more overweight."

The number one reason people overeat is because of stress.

The number one reason people go on vacation is to get away from stress. And what do we do when we go on vacation?

We eat and drink a lot of alcohol.

Everyone Will Tell You How to Lose Weight

In doing research for my first book, *Discover Your Thinner Self*, I was overwhelmed and inundated with the amount of information available for weight loss. Thousands and thousands of books have been written about diet, nutrition, fitness, and exercise. There are more than 50,000 books available on Amazon pertaining to diet, weight loss, health, fitness, and nutrition. At the grocery store checkout, you'll see hundreds and hundreds of magazine articles written about weight loss, many of them touted on the front cover. There are numerous weight loss programs advertised on TV and radio such as Weight Watchers, Jenny Craig, Nutrisystem, The South Beach Diet, The Atkins Diet, and many more. Not to mention the other types of diets such as the Keto diet, Paleo diet, Mediterranean diet, etc.

With all the information out there about dieting, who or what do you believe and act on? How do you choose? One expert will tell you one thing, another will say just the opposite. For example, should you eat breakfast or not?

That depends on who you believe. Most weight loss and diet books and programs suggest that eating a healthy breakfast high in protein will help you lose weight. They all state "it's backed by research."

Harvey Diamond, Author of *Fit for Life*, one of the best-selling books of all time, tells you to only eat fruits before noon. Still, another opinion by Paul and Patricia Bragg is not to eat breakfast. Paul & Patricia Bragg are health and nutrition experts. Paul is credited with opening the first health food store in the U.S. and taught many celebrities including Jack LaLanne, Clint Eastwood, and Gloria Swanson. You've probably seen Bragg Apple Cider Vinegar at your grocery or health food store.

What I learned is there are many misconceptions and false beliefs about weight loss and dieting. A misconception is a view or opinion that is incorrect because it is based on false evidence, faulty thinking, or understanding.

My goal in writing this book is to help you sort out the myths from the facts and to be your guide along your weight-loss journey. Rick Frishman, Best-selling author, publisher, and speaker, usually tells his audience at his *Author 101University* workshops, "A book can change a person's life." It is my sincere hope that this book might improve your life.

As with everything, there are a few rules. I have only two:

The First Rule is: Don't believe a word I say.

Why do I say that? Because it's my experience from which I'm speaking. Each of us is unique and different. We have different eating preferences, different habits, different body chemistry. What might work for me might not work for you. What might work for you, might not work for someone else. Just because a "Diet" worked for your neighbor doesn't mean it will work for you.

That, however, doesn't make what I'm about to share with you true or false, right or wrong. It just makes it based on my experience.

To successfully reduce weight and, more importantly, keep it off, there are some universal laws of nature that must be adhered to. These will be discussed throughout the book.

The Second Rule is that you "Be Open."

I ask you to keep an open mind about the information being presented. That does not mean that what I'm going to teach you is right or wrong. It just means it worked for me. Whatever is working for you, great, keep doing it. Whatever doesn't work, toss out. I will share with you what works for me and has worked for others. All I ask is you keep an open mind.

Mark Twain said: "It ain't what you don't know that gets you into trouble; it's what you know for sure that just ain't so." Be careful of what you think you might know about losing weight because it might not be accurate. Worse, it could be detrimental to your health.

Have you noticed I've asked a lot of questions?

Are you are annoyed with reading so many questions?

I don't ask them to annoy you or treat you like a 5-year-old. The reason I ask a lot of questions is that learning requires energy. I also ask questions to keep you engaged because it's been proven to help you retain more of what you're taught. It's important to think about your answers to the questions being asked because pondering them might reveal some insight about yourself you might not be aware of now.

Throughout this book, I will repeat certain things because experts have determined that if you hear or read something more than once, you're more likely to remember it. While *what* you're learning is important, it is also important *how* it's being taught.

Many of you, like me, probably have forgotten much of what we learned. That's why many of you fail to do what you once knew. Samuel Johnson said, "We often need to be reminded more than we need to be instructed." Often the key to growth, progress, and success is not having to learn anything new, you just need to be reminded about what you once learned so that you can consistently do that which you know.

Today, there are many people who'd rather suffer the consequences of poor health, chronic illnesses, major medical ailments such as cancer or Type 2 diabetes or even death rather than give up their bad eating habits to lose weight. Can you relate to this? Hopefully not, which is why your reading this book.

The average weight loss for contestants on *The Biggest Loser* is 127 pounds. Over time, the average contestant regained 66 percent of the weight they lost. In other words, they regained 83 pounds. A few gained more than they initially lost.

Americans are Getting Fatter

Socially acceptable body weight is increasing. Why? Because individuals are content with their weight. They are not aware their lifestyles are killing them or that being overweight has severe health-related consequences. They are less motivated to shed those unhealthy pounds now. Let's face it, it's easier to keep eating the same unhealthy fast foods and snacking on junk food than to prepare healthy, nutritious snacks.

Many of you also avoid exercising or doing any physical activity. Today, both kids and adults would rather sit and play video games on their phones, tablets, or computers than move around. Virtual reality technology is replacing many sports such as tennis. You can play tennis with a professional without going to the tennis court.

Let's face it, it takes less effort to keep doing the same thing than to make a complete lifestyle change. Reducing weight is so hard that many people simply don't want to make any effort whatsoever. Good intentions are ineffective and meaningless.

We all intend to lose weight. We all want to lose weight. Well, maybe most of us. But I'm certain you do want to achieve a healthy weight and maintain it. Until you act and commit to shedding your unwanted and unhealthy pounds, nothing will happen. Would you agree with me that nothing about your eating habits will change unless you do something different?

Bestselling author, Dr. David Friedman, in his international award-winning number one best-selling book, *Food Sanity* stated, "Whoever snuck the "S" in FAST FOOD was a clever marketer. The chemicals that fast food restaurants use have been linked to many health ailments including obesity." Too often it's easier and more convenient to pick up a meal at the drive-thru than to take the time to prepare a healthy meal at home. Once this happens, for many of you, like me, the desire to lose weight is kaput. Out the door, gone. We feel guilty for cheating on our diet. We give up and revert to our old eating habits.

If you want to grasp the concept of what extra weight is doing to your body, try this simple exercise. Carry a one-gallon jug of water in each hand for as long as you can. A one-gallon jug of water weighs approximately 8.36 pounds. In other words, you're lugging around almost 17 pounds of extra weight. After you put the jugs of water down, notice how much lighter you feel. Imagine how much better you'd feel if you lost 20 pounds.

You need to stay conscious of your own weight and the consequences of excess weight because, as I noted above, self-perceptions are changing because it is so common to be overweight or obese. So many people are overweight that we lose perspective. You see so many other people heavier than you that you think you're fine because you're thinner. You're wrong. You're both overweight.

That's a consequence of America's obesity epidemic: the perception of what is normal has shifted.

That reminds me of a story. Some friends were having dinner with us one evening. John mentioned he was going to attend his fiftieth class reunion. He and his kids had just finished browsing through his high school yearbook when one of the kids said, "Hey, dad, can we see that again?"

"Sure why?" John replied.

His son opened the yearbook and flipped through it. As the pages cascaded, his son pointed out an interesting observation. "Dad, did you notice that all your high school classmates were thin? There aren't any fat kids."

"No, not really."

Lyle chimed in, "Now that I think about it, there weren't any overweight kids in my high school either."

Afterward, I went back home to look through my high school yearbook. Wow, what a revelation. There were only a handful of heavy-set kids, none whom I would consider overweight.

Yet, today, many children in grades K through 12 are overweight, some are obese. Think about how that affects self-perception. Sometimes it takes someone to point out the obvious.

Can you relate to this story?

Unfortunately, overweight or obese adults incorrectly believe that their body weight is just fine. It's a vicious cycle. As more individuals become obese, more of them are fine with being overweight, they see others with larger bodies, and they become less motivated to shed the extra pounds. Being overweight is the new normal.

In this politically correct society, many people believe you shouldn't do or say anything to make overweight people feel uncomfortable. Even physicians walk a fine line. They don't want patients to have unhealthy bodies but haven't figured out how to make them understand they need to get rid of weight without offending or appearing insensitive.

Today's doctors don't want to intervene. The amount of effort required to understand the patient's needs for weight reduction is more than many doctors are willing to put forth. Instead, they're content to write you prescriptions for medication and manage symptoms rather than address your underlying issues. It's much easier and more profitable for them to prescribe medication than take the time to help a person change their lifestyle.

Some of these same physicians are overweight themselves and don't see a need to help their patients.

While vacationing with my wife in Costa Rica, I met an overweight doctor we'll call Randy. He boasted that most of his patients weighed 300 to 400 pounds.

He had to shed 80 pounds before his orthopedic surgeon would do his hip replacement because he had too much fat. He was still

100 pounds overweight. In other words, Randy weighed 180 pounds more than what is considered healthy.

Randy began to tell me that when you get to be his age, money wasn't as important as lifestyle. I looked at Randy and said, "I understand."

To which Randy replied, "How could you, you're nowhere near my age."

"Yes, I am," I retorted.

Randy said, "I'm 58. How old are you?"

I replied, "63."

Randy shook his head and walked away. That was the last time I saw him.

Approximately 61 percent of nurses in the U.S. are overweight or clinically obese. And we wonder why there's an epidemic of people being overweight? Perhaps we should listen to Robert Kiyosaki who said, "Stop taking advice from people more messed up than you."

Can I share a horse story with you?

Great!

A few years ago, while in Las Vegas, I met the owner of a "prized" thoroughbred racehorse. During our conversation, he explained to me how he made certain his horse got the best nutritional supplements and ate the healthiest food to optimize the horse's performance. He boasted how he hired the best licensed and certified veterinarian to thoroughly examine the horse each week. He bragged how the horse got the best dental care available.

The horse had his own personal trainer to exercise it every day. He made sure that the horse's environment was optimal for social interaction to keep the horse's spirits up. No expense was spared on maintaining the horse's health so the horse could perform at its best. Indeed, the man's knowledge about what the horse needed, and was provided, for optimal performance was remarkable.

But what made the biggest impression on me meeting this owner was how he cared for himself. You see, this gentleman was at least 75 pounds overweight. When the waiter served the owner's lunch, it was a huge hamburger loaded with cheese, bacon, lettuce and tomato, ketchup, mustard, and mayo. Of course, there was a side of golden French fries and an ice-cold Coke to wash down the food. It was apparent and obvious that this owner was more concerned about the health and care of his racehorse than himself.

Pushing the conversation, I asked the owner how often he'd get a check-up from his doctor. The owner scoffed at the idea. His response, "I haven't been to a doctor in years. I'm as healthy as a horse." *Uh-huh*, I thought.

Now I'm certain you are thinking, I don't own a prized racehorse so what's this got to do with me? Sadly, probably more than you realize. Do you own a pet, such as a dog or a cat? If you do, you most likely, like so many others, feed your dogs and pets more carefully than your own kids or yourself.

It's time to re-evaluate your health and fitness philosophy. There's a reason for the statement, "…is as healthy as a horse." Now is the time you should care for yourself like a prized racehorse so you can perform at your best. Wouldn't you like to have more energy? Feel better? Look better? Be able to be more active with your kids and grandkids? If not, you need not read any further because this is not the right book for you.

That Food You Crave Isn't Just Food

I'm of the opinion that food manufacturers are working in tandem with big pharma. You'll learn how some food additives started out based on research for new drugs. It's scary to think that research for new drugs is how chemical compounds are now food additives.

Like certain drugs, many processed foods are addicting. Researchers found that Oreos are more addicting than cocaine. It's unimaginable that a cookie is more addictive than an illegal drug. Do you have a hard time eating only one or two Oreos?

Do you crave potato chips? When they say "Betcha can't eat just one," it's not a dare. It's a fact! I know because I'd eat an entire canister of Pringles at one time. I couldn't stop myself. Now I know the reason why.

In 1995 the average grocery store carried about 15,000 products. Today, it's over 50,000. Now, I don't know about you, but

I haven't heard of that many new fruits, vegetables or berries being discovered during this time.

We're All Sensitive About Weight

Intervention is problematic because weight is such a sensitive issue for most people.

After all, how many men feel awkward if their wives or girlfriends ask, "Does this make me look fat?" If the husband or boyfriend is truthful, the woman's feelings are hurt. It's easier to not be honest and tell her, "You look great." The smart answer is "Do I look Stupid?"

Unfortunately, the wives and girlfriends probably are also afraid to say anything about their man's expanding waistline.

Thankfully, my doctor didn't care about being politically correct or perceived as being insensitive. He flat out told me, "Lose weight or find a new doctor because you'll die."

Everyone wants a
- "Magic pill,"
- "Secret formula," or
- "Special food" to produce extraordinary weight-loss results.

The most sought-after solution is often the newest, fastest fat buster available that doesn't require dieting and exercise. I'm here to tell you, there is no miraculous fruit, vegetable, berry, or supplement to reduce weight. Don't bother looking for it. It doesn't exist. If it did, we'd all be thinner.

There are no shortcuts to weight reduction and a healthier lifestyle.

There is no lotion to rub on your belly to get rid of the fat.

There are no products that produce instant results. There's no genie in a bottle to grant you a wish of being thinner and healthier.

Here's the good news. You can reduce weight without having to:
- Order special foods or products
- Follow an exercise program
- Follow restrictive recipes
- Count calories or do food exchanges
- Undergo surgeries, or

- Take herbs, teas or pills

So, what is the best way to attain a healthy weight and be able to maintain it? It's not by dieting because diets are generally extreme, unhealthy, expensive, and temporary.

The fact remains that you must choose to make a conscious decision for a lifestyle change. Without changing your eating behaviors, you won't create new habits. Without new eating habits, if you do shed a few pounds, most likely you'll regain all the weight you lost, and in some cases, even more.

According to Dr. David Katz, M.D., who refers to Michael Pollan, a simple solution to reduce weight in a healthy and sustainable manner is to…

- Eat holistic food
- Not too much
- Mostly plants
- Avoid processed foods, and
- Drink lots of pure water

I'd add one more to Dr. Katz's list: Get adequate sleep.

Simple yes? But, not so easy to do. If it were, we'd all be thinner and healthier.

Unfortunately, most of us have a SAD food intake. SAD, which stands for Standard American Diet, is the primary cause of chronic disease and illness. But, no matter how much proof or evidence exists on the health benefits of eating a mostly plant-based diet, the fact remains that most Americans will never give up their processed foods and SAD, fast food, lifestyle.

"You can't work out (exercise away) bad eating habits."
Robert W. Jones, Network Together Founder

Lose Weight One Pound at a Time

Did you know, the word "Diet" is derived from the Greek word "Diaita" meaning "A way of living?" Food used to be consumed as fuel for the body. Today, however, it's used for comfort, to deal with stress and enjoyment.

Here's some more good news. You don't have to worry about losing all the unwanted and unhealthy weight at one time. You just needed to lose a little bit at a time. You can reach a healthy weight that is easy to maintain by choosing to reduce your weight one ounce and one pound at a time.

You see, you gained weight one pound at a time. You didn't gain it all at once or overnight. It's like eating an elephant, not literally, of course.

So, how do you eat an elephant?

One bite at a time.

Likewise, you can lose weight one ounce and one pound at a time, That's the power of little, seemingly inconsequential improvements to your daily eating habits. It's the smallest changes to your eating habits and lifestyle done consistently over a long time (more than 90 days) that can make the biggest difference to achieving a healthy weight and, more importantly, keep it off.

Darren Hardy described weight loss in his book, *The Compound Effect*. He talks about three buddies who grew up together. They all lived in the same neighborhood. They're all married and have average health and body weight. Friend one, called Larry, plods along doing what he's always done. He's happy, or so he thinks but complains occasionally and nothing much ever changes.

Friend two, Scott, starts making small, seemingly inconsequential, positive changes. He begins reading 10 pages of a good book each day, cuts 125 calories from his diet, drinks pure water instead of soda. He also starts walking about a mile each day. Easy stuff anyone can do.

Friend three, Brad, makes a few poor choices. He buys a big screen TV and watches more programs. He watches the Food Channel trying out new recipes, cheesy casseroles, and desserts. He also installs a bar in his home and added one more alcoholic beverage per week.

At the end of five months, no perceivable differences exist between the three friends. No noticeable differences at the end of 12 months. But, at the end of 18 months, measurable differences start showing up. Within 25 months (a little over two years) you can see big differences between the three.

Scott has lost 33 pounds. Brad has gained 34 pounds; Brad weighs 67 pounds more than Scott.

There are other more significant differences.

Scott is doing very well at work, received a promotion, and his marriage is thriving. Brad's unhappy at work, his marriage is on the rocks, and he is miserable.

Larry is pretty much exactly where he was two years earlier.

Would you like to be 20, 30, or 40 pounds lighter by this time next year?

Keep in mind, if you shed just one-half pound each week, you'll have lost 26 pounds in a year. Another way to think about it is if you lose just three pounds a month, in a year you will have dropped 36 pounds. I believe that you can lose two to three pounds per month. Would you agree with me that's certainly doable? Of course, it is.

Charles Duhigg in his book, *The Power of Habit,* spoke about keystone habits. A keystone habit is changing one habit that can change your entire life because it has a ripple effect.

As an example, if you drink soda or diet soda, switch to drinking pure water. If you don't like water, figure out a way to add natural flavor like lemon, orange, watermelon, cucumber, pineapple, or other fruits and berries to give it a delicious, thirst-quenching taste.

Researchers found more than 70 percent of the U.S. population suffers from chronic dehydration. Drink more *pure* water.

Folks, our bodies are made up of 60 percent water.

Do you drink a minimum of 64 ounces of pure water each day?

Did you know that much of the time you when you think you're hungry, you're thirsty?

This could be one reason most of us eat too much. We should be drinking more *pure* water.

What do I mean by pure water?

Pure water, in my opinion, is distilled water, water processed by reverse osmosis, or spring water. It is not the processed flavored waters. There is debate and dispute as to which is better between distilled water, reverse osmosis water, and spring water. You choose which is best for you. We'll delve into the water controversy in greater detail in the next chapter.

Avoid diet soda because it causes weight gain. I can hear you now. "But, it's zero calories." Yes, it's zero calories, but it contains the artificial sweetener aspartame. According to Dr. Joseph Mercola, research shows that Aspartame slows your metabolism and prevents your body from absorbing vitamins, minerals, and nutrients. Thus, your body is starving and goes into starvation mode. Starvation mode is when your body fights like heck to keep the fat on.

So, what can you do to attain a healthy weight?

To achieve a permanent healthy weight, you must make lifestyle changes. Here's what I know. I can share some inspiring new ideas with you, give you a great tip or insight to attaining a healthy weight. And, I might be able to change your mind about your ideas about eating healthy. But you cannot change your life until you change your eating behaviors. Behaviors done consistently over time such that they become new habits.

No one can order or command you to change your eating behaviors. All I ask is that you be open to doing it for yourself.

Permanent behavior is the key to lasting change, but not behavior changed once or for a short stint. After all, how many diets did you start that did not last? Permanent behavior equals habit. Losing weight and being able to keep it off is not like getting a vaccination. You don't get one shot and forget about it. It doesn't work that way.

Now, you might be asking, "How do I form these new habits?"

Hey, that's a great question.

According to researchers, a behavior needs to be repeated, it must be consistent and done long enough to form a habit.

The problem is the consistent and long part of that equation.

Can you relate to that?

Probably you can because that's where everybody screws up. But here's how to fix that. For a new behavior to happen consistently you must find a way to remove all thinking, all discipline, and all willpower from the equation. If you need to rely on any of that, you're screwed. Have you experienced a lack of willpower or discipline? Yeah, if you are being honest, you have, as seen from all your past-resolutions, diets, and failed promises.

To succeed in replacing a new habit in place of a bad habit, you'll want to tie your new behavior to an existing habit. Something you already do automatically without thinking or needing to have discipline or willpower. For instance, brushing your teeth first thing in the morning. Once you've finished brushing your teeth, drink a glass of pure water immediately afterward. Later in this book, you'll be given more ideas and suggestions you can apply for a day, a week, and a month.

You'll see that these small, seemingly inconsequential positive improvements done consistently over an extended time compound to give you noticeable results and lasting change.

One of the most asked questions is, "How much should I weigh?" or "What is my ideal weight?"

The simple answer is there is no ideal weight.

Unfortunately, too many people rely on a body mass index (BMI) as a method to determine a perfect weight. Body mass index measures a person's height in relation to their weight, but it is not a perfect measurement.

Research has demonstrated errors occur attempting to identify a normal weight range.

Your ideal weight depends on several factors such as your body composition, height, age, weight, frame size, gender, bone density, body fat distribution, and muscle-to-fat ratio.

Further, BMI fails to indicate a person's healthiness and overall well-being. As an example, just because a person is thin does not mean they are healthy. A thin person might appear fit, but they might be ill and suffering from poor eating habits, a drug issue, or a fad diet lacking in proper nutrition. Nor is it a good indicator for cardiovascular disease.

In February of 2017, Bob Harper, the fitness idol from *The Biggest Loser*, suffered a near-fatal heart attack while working out at the gym. It seems unfathomable that Harper would be susceptible to a heart attack. But, as he learned, being healthy is more than being fit and trim. It's about balance and providing your body with proper nutrition.

The BMI doesn't distinguish between a couch potato and a bodybuilder. While BMI is good to study population obesity statistics, it should never be used for determining an individual's overall fitness.

Even the mathematician Adolphe Quetelet, who created the formula used for the BMI, warned against using it as an indicator for an individual's health. More than 50 million Americans have been inaccurately labeled as obese or overweight based on BMI.

According to Dr. Mehmet Oz, generally, as a rule, your waist size should be one-half of your height. In other words, if you're 5'8" (68 inches), your waist should be 34" or less. If you're 6'0" (72 inches) your waist should be 36.

There are many misconceptions about reducing weight. One of these is that eating more fresh fruits, vegetables, and berries will help reduce weight. Eating more fruits and vegetables is not a secret to reducing weight nor does it guarantee dropping unwanted pounds. It is true that consuming more fruits, vegetables, and berries is a key component to shedding weight. But several studies conducted on the impact of eating more fruits and vegetables alone found it had no impact on losing weight.

Many so-called weight-loss experts advocate a high protein low or no carbohydrate diet for weight loss. Since his heart attack, Bob Harper changed his diet from a high protein, low fat, low carbs to a more balanced approach that includes "good" carbs from vegetables, fruits, and whole grains.

Keep in mind there are different types of protein used for different purposes. Confused? You should be because how often to you see an advertisement for protein to add weight and build muscle? Yet, protein is also touted for weight loss at the same time. So, which is it – to lose weight or to gain weight? The answer is, it depends. Again, depending on what you're trying to accomplish will determine which protein you should consume.

Another misconception is that eating only salads will help you to lose weight. Eating a salad at every meal will not help you lose weight either because some salads, in fact, have more calories than a regular, balanced meal. Salad items can cause a person to consume a higher number of calories and saturated fats than they realize. For instance, many dressings are oil based. A teaspoon of oil has 45 calories and 5g of fat. Other culprits are bacon, cheese, and croutons. A better alternative is to use lemon juice or salsa as a low calorie, low-fat dressing. Or, make your own vinaigrette with olive oil, apple cider vinegar, and thyme and other spices.

Many people incorrectly believe that it costs too much to eat healthy. Eating healthier, however, doesn't have to cost a lot of money. The truth of the matter is healthy foods are often less expensive than fast foods. Last time I checked, a meal at McDonald's, Burger King, Wendy's, or Panda Express cost more than seven dollars per person. Research has shown that choosing nutritious foods purchased from the supermarket can save consumers money.

The real issue is many individuals do not want to make the time or effort to prepare a nutritious dish and prefer the convenience of the McDonald's drive-thru window or to pick-up a bucket of KFC chicken.

Can you relate to this?

If this is one of your excuses, it's time to decide how committed and determined you are to get rid of your excess fat.

The average fast food meal costs upwards of six dollars, and closer to eight dollars. Combo or extra value meals should be avoided because they tend to have more calories than you need in one course. It is also prudent to limit the use of toppings that are high in fat and calories such as bacon, cheese, mayonnaise, or tartar sauce. Instead of drinking soda or sweetened beverages, sip on water. Whenever possible, choose steamed or baked items over fried ones.

Another mistaken belief is that fresh foods are healthier than frozen or canned foods. Frozen or canned foods provide as many nutrients as fresh ones, but at a lower cost. Read the nutrition facts label. Healthy options include low-salt veggies and fruits packed in their own juice or water without added sugar. Canned tuna packed in water is easy to store and won't break the budget. If, however, you're going to have tuna, do so without the mayo.

Avoid crash diets because they are unhealthy and unsustainable. What this means for you is that while you'll lose weight, you won't be able to keep it off. Remember, diets are just a temporary fix that doesn't address the underlying issues. There are several programs that claim an individual can lose 10 pounds within two weeks. This is partially true. A person can shed as much as 10 pounds, or more, on a crash diet within two weeks.

The problem arises if you don't adjust or modify your eating behavior and lifestyle. Once you resume your normal eating habits, the weight will return. All you will have done is deplete your body of important nutrients and burn muscle.

Skipping meals might seem like the fastest way to lose weight, but it doesn't work that way. Missing meals will not help you lose weight. When you skip meals, your body goes into starvation mode and you retain weight. Your body panics. The panic causes the body to store fat and makes it more difficult to burn off.

Skipping one meal occasionally won't hurt you but starving yourself daily will. Further, skipping a meal can lead to bingeing or excessive eating later. It makes you hungrier, causing you to eat more at the next meal.

People ask me, "How did you lose your weight so fast?" I used HCG. HCG is a hormone from a pregnant woman that you inject into your belly. I do **not** recommend using HCG to reduce weight.

Are you curious as to why I wouldn't recommend something that worked for me?

Here's the reason. When you're using HCG, you are on 550 calories per day for six weeks. After that, you're on 1,250 calories for another six weeks. That is not a lot of calories. Many meals served at restaurants have more than 1,500 calories. Also, 90 percent of those who do lose weight using HCG gain it all back, some even more. You are not taught to modify your eating behaviors. It is a temporary solution. I was fortunate to do research and understand the importance of modifying my eating behaviors and habits.

That reminds me of a story about my friend Jerry. Jerry wanted to lose weight the same time I did. He was going to show me that I didn't need to be on HCG or pay a doctor. He was right, but with different results.

Jerry chose not to eat. He'd eat one meal, lunch, every other day. The other day he just drank water and a coke. Jerry did this for approximately eight weeks, nearly two months. Jerry lost over 40 pounds.

However, one day while driving, he looked at me and showed me his arm. "Does your skin hang like this?" he asked.

"No."

"Well how come mine is like this?"

"Because you lost muscle mass instead of fat. You starved yourself."

To which Jerry responded, "You don't know what you're talking about. I'm going to the gym and workout."

A few weeks later, Jerry asked me, "Can you lift more than fifteen pounds?"

"Of course," I said. "Why do you ask?"

"Because I can't."

"Well, what does your trainer say? I asked.

"He asked if I was eating. I told him 'No. I want to lose weight.' He said I need to eat because I'm burning muscle instead of fat."

Since then Jerry has resumed eating. He is regaining his muscle tone and doing great.

The lesson is that if you don't provide your body with proper fuel and nourishment you could do damage to yourself. What are your views on food? Do you think of it as fuel for your body?

Strive for lasting results by achieving a healthy weight in a healthy and sustainable manner. There are no instant solutions. Fad diets and pills to lose weight are extreme and temporary. Excessive calorie restrictions can lead to loss of muscle rather than fat. If the body does not get enough energy, it will begin to breakdown muscle tissue for fuel. Muscle burns more calories than fat does. If the weight returns, it is usually fat. The fat reduces the body's ability to burn calories. Thereby causing an increase in weight. My suggestion is to concentrate more on how your clothes fit instead of what the scale reads.

Have you been told that eating before bed will cause you to gain weight or not make you fat? Again, this is a partial truth.

Certain foods will cause you to gain weight if consumed late at night, while others can help with weight loss. The point is to be careful when inhaling a late-night snack.

If possible, avoid eating after 7:00 p.m. More about this will be discussed in Chapter Four.

There are some health professionals and weight-loss clinics that advocate a person doesn't need to be highly motivated to start a weight-loss regimen. They only need to begin.

This is partly accurate. To demonstrate my point, consider how many people start the new year with a resolution to lose weight. Of those, 80 percent or more will quit within 30 days, if not sooner.

Researchers have found that those with a compelling reason to reduce weight are more successful. To be successful at reducing weight you must be determined, dedicated, and committed. It's not so much about starting or wanting to lose weight, as its being compelled to follow through. People start diets all the time but never stick with it.

They give up after a few days, weeks, or months. Lack of commitment and determination is the main reason people fail to lose weight. January resolutions without a high motivation to drop those unwanted pounds are unlikely to succeed.

Once you decide to reduce your weight, commit to it. Then act! Because the universe will conspire to make it happen.

In addition, changing your relationship with food and how you view it can have a significant influence on weight loss. If you consider food as fuel for your body, you'll most likely consume less than if it is used for comfort.

Get a support team to keep you stay accountable because it will vastly help you along your weight-reduction journey. Consider attending group meetings because researchers have found that those who attend meetings on a regular basis tend to lose up to three times as much weight compared to those who don't attend. As I mentioned before, losing weight is hard, especially if you do it alone. It is better to have a support team. Find someone to keep you accountable. We all have reasons to justify putting off reducing weight.

There is not a perfect time to start to reduce weight. I know about these excuses. I used them all. I accomplished shedding 50 pounds in four months that I failed to do anytime during the prior eight years.

When trying to reduce weight or just maintaining it, people generally think about calories and grams of carbs. What they forget is the grams of sugar. Especially processed sugar. A Starbucks Grande (that's the medium size drink) Java Chip Frappuccino has 66g of sugar in it. Not to be outdone, the Starbucks Grande S'mores Frappuccino has 68g of sugar. Based on a 2,000 calorie/day diet, a person should consume about 50g of sugar. That means just having one of the popular drinks at Starbucks gives you more sugar than you need in an entire day!

Be careful of making exceptions; they tend to become the rule. Have you heard this before, "Go ahead, have just one?" "One cookie won't hurt you. One piece of candy won't hurt you. It won't kill you." No! It won't kill you. No! It won't hurt you. But it will prevent you from losing weight.

It's not what you do when someone is watching, it's what you do when you're alone and no one is watching. Do you sneak snacks when you're alone? Stop doing that. You're only lying to yourself. If you feel you need to snack, call a friend. Go for a walk. Do something other than giving in to that craving. Other suggestions and ideas are included in Appendix A.

Here are three tips you can start to use today if you choose to improve your eating habits.

- Substitute pure water for sodas (soft drinks), juices, or flavored water. Drink more pure water.
- Avoid or reduce your alcohol consumption.
- Eat off a blue salad plate. Blue is an appetite suppressant, whereas, red and yellow are appetite stimulants. That's probably why McDonald's, Denny's, Wendy's, Burger King, KFC, and other fast food places use red and yellow in their color schemes.

Also, by eating off a smaller plate, you'll reduce your food consumption and it will seem like you're eating more.

You need to get adequate sleep to successfully reduce weight. The average person who is sleep deprived will consume an extra 500 calories per day. It takes an average of reducing 500 calories per day for an entire week to lose one pound. Think about that. You're going in the wrong direction without adequate sleep.

You must eat slower to reduce weight. Put your fork or spoon down between bites. Stop using them like a shovel. This will be discussed in more detail in Chapter Four.

If you want results to attain a healthy weight and keep it, keep reading.

No matter what, you must put in the time, effort, and work to attain a healthy weight.

There is no amount of money you can pay someone to lose your weight. They can't eat for you. They can't exercise for you. They can't drink lots of water each day for you. And they certainly, can't take the proper nutrition for you.

You have the power to choose to make better decisions. You can choose to transform your lifestyle to improve your health.

The only question is: will you choose to do so? Or will you be another statistic?

What will be your weight story?

Once you start to implement the ideas set forth, it's important to debrief. If you can, find someone reading this book and connect with them. If not, ask yourself these four questions:

1. What happened during the week?
2. How did it make you feel? Did you have an aha moment?
3. What did you learn from the events during the week?
4. How can you use the information going forward?

Is There Some Magic to be Found in 90 Days?

There is none. Zero. Zip. When I say you can create a healthy lifestyle in 90 days, I don't mean to suggest you can reach your goal weight or change your life in that time. But you can change some habits. Not all of them, of course, but some. And it's important because change is a choice. You need to choose new behaviors, one at a time, and practice, practice, practice until those choices are new behaviors and habits. The Tao Te Ching says, "Confront the difficult while it is still easy; accomplish the great task by a series of small acts."

This book is full of suggestions and choices and options. I write about new ways to eat, new things to try, new ways of talking to yourself. Try some. I guarantee that if you choose to change your life and try out and implement these little changes, one at a time and consistently, you will be on your way to changing your lifestyle in 90 days. What do you have to lose (besides those extra pounds you're lugging around)?

Redemption to Good Health

Redemption to good health begins with getting your emotional, psychological, and mental attitude aligned before the physical. Because any weight reduction journey begins with being mentally, emotionally, and psychologically ready. It's mental belief. If you don't believe you can do it, you won't.

It's not what others believe about you, it's what you believe about yourself. And, it doesn't matter if what you believe is true of not. It only matters that you believe it's true.

Chapter 2

The Shocking Truth About Water

Water, water everywhere, not a drop to drink.
"Rime of the Ancient Mariner"
by Samuel Taylor Coleridge

If you're having trouble losing weight or keeping it off, the food you eat might not be to blame. Maybe, just maybe, the culprit is the water you're drinking to wash down the food you're eating.

Is the water you're drinking safe? Are you sure?

Because there could be contaminants in your drinking water that have been connected to gut issues, weight gain, food intolerance, autoimmune disease, and cancer.

In 1993, a legal clerk named Erin Brockovich received national media attention when she exposed the Pacific Gas and Electric Company (PG&E) in California for contaminating the water supply in Hinkley, California. PG&E was exposed for contaminating the groundwater and ponds near Hinkley with chromium 6 and other toxic chemicals. This tainted water caused liver damage, reproductive issues, birth defects, and cancer to the people living in Hinkley.

Academy award-winning actress Julia Roberts portrayed Erin Brockovich in the critically acclaimed film. Despite the negative exposure and publicity and a $333 million class action settlement in 1996, the problem still exists in 2019. And, it's gotten worse. When most Americans drink tap water, they're also getting a dose of industrial or agricultural waste products connected to cancer, brain, and nervous system damage, fertility problems, hormonal disruption, and child-development deficiencies.

As of July of 2017, chromium 6 had been found in more than 250 million (250,000,000) homes in all 50 states. This is the disturbing truth documented by EWG's Tap Water Database, the most comprehensive and complete source available on the quality of the U.S. drinking water, collecting and analyzing data from approximately 50,000 public water utilities.

According to Dr. David Friedman, "It's ironic that people will spend more money on organic vegetables and fruits believing they are safer to eat. It's ironic because if you buy your organic produce from a grocery store, watch for about an hour and see how much water is sprayed on them. More than likely, the water used to spray these beautiful, organic produce is from contaminated tap water. It kind of defeats the purpose doesn't it?"

The bulk of the U.S. drinking water supply gets a passing grade from federal and state regulatory agencies. The Environmental Protection Agency (EPA) labels many of the contaminants in our water "within safe limits." Here's the fallacy. The average person drinks one to two glasses of water each day. More than 70 percent of the U.S. population suffers from dehydration. But, others, like me, drink eight to ten glasses of water each day. What this means is if your neighbor next door drinks one to two glasses of water per day and you're drinking ten glasses, you're drinking five times as much water as your neighbor. Do you really feel it's fair for the EPA to say that toxic chemicals in your water are "within safe limits?"

Keep in mind that many of these toxic chemicals, such as Perfluorooctanoic Acid (PFOA) and Perfluorooctanoic Sulfonate (PFOS), accumulate in the body every time you consume them. Perfluoroalkyl substances are *not* naturally found in the environment. In other words, these are man-made contaminants. They are used for making such things as waterproof materials, paper packaging, fabrics, grease, and stain resistant products, and firefighting foam.

What happens after consuming these "within safe limits" chemicals after two years? After five years? Or, after ten years? Remember what Darren Hardy said about the compound effect of seemingly inconsequential habits that done consistently over a long period of time?

They will give you noticeable results. In this case, drinking the water containing chemicals within seemingly inconsequential "safe limits" consistently over a long period of time will result in you contracting chronic diseases and illnesses. We just don't know what we don't know about these chemicals building up in our bodies until it's too late. Research suggests that continued exposure to low levels of PFOA in drinking water may result in harmful health effects.

Water Quality Association Deputy Executive Director Pauli Undesser said, "It is important for consumers to know that public water systems are *not* required to test and monitor for PFOA and PFOS." Still not convinced your water might not be contaminated. The EPA has not added a new contaminant to the list of regulated drinking water pollutants in more than 20 years. What this means for you is that there are no legal limits for more than 160 unregulated pollutants the tests detect in the nation's tap water.

A study published in the February 13, 2018 edition of PLOS Medicine found that those with a greater amount of Perfluoroalkyl compounds (PFASs) concentrations in their systems regained more weight, especially in women. The data illustrated a potential for PFAS to interfere with human body weight regulation and metabolism. Participants in the study might have been exposed to the PFAS through contaminated food packaging.

What gives the EPA the right to pretend they have the knowledge to determine exactly what amount of deadly chemicals you can drink before it's considered a concern or detriment to your health? Ronald Reagan said that the nine words people fear the most is, "I'm from the government and I'm here to help." Now you know why people fear government involvement.

The EWG found that the quality of drinking water can greatly vary based on income and the geographic area it comes from. For example, water tests in Topeka, Kansas found four pesticides used on corn fields in the drinking water. The Des Moines Water Works in Iowa fights daily to control the level of nitrates and other chemicals used in local farming. It's not just from farm areas either. The East Los Angeles Water District detected the most contaminants of concern with 14 different pollutants above established health guidelines in its 2015 water test. The district serves 115,000 people whose household income is more than 20 percent below the national average.

By contrast, the water system for Merrick, New York, which serves about 117,000 citizens on Long Island, is one of the cleanest in the nation. The median household income in Merrick is more than two-and-a-half times the national average.

There is a scene at the end of the James Bond movie *Quantum of Solace* where James Bond, played by Daniel Craig, watches another agent pour a glass of water for one of the villains from what appears to be a harmless water bottle. The water is the water contaminated by the villain with their illegal dumping of industrial toxic waste. What's important about this scene in a James Bond movie? Because in the summer of 2015, high levels of lead were found in the drinking water of Flint, Michigan. The water was deemed safe to drink by federal and state regulators. The contaminated water was discovered only because a worried mother contacted the Environmental Protection Agency (EPA) after her child got sick.

More than 250-plus contaminants were detected in water samples that are considered perfectly legal under the Safe Drinking Water Act or state regulations. However, the level of these 250-plus contaminants are above levels scientific studies have found to cause health risks. So, let me be clear about this. The government tells you water that contains more than 250 toxic chemicals is safe to drink, but there is scientific evidence that the same water causes health risks. And we wonder why chronic diseases and illnesses are on the rise.

If you think buying bottled water is safe, think again. Americans spend almost $17 billion each year on bottled water believing it's safe. According to Dr. David Friedman, B.S., N.D., D.C., author of the international award-winning, number one bestselling book, *Food Sanity,* and host of *To Your Good Health Radio* on Radio MD Podcast, the federal government does more testing and quality control on tap water than on bottled water.

Not surprisingly, the bottled water industry disagrees with the assertion that bottled water is regulated less rigorously than tap water. Stephen Kay, of the International Bottled Water Association, asserts that bottled water in the United States is regulated as a packaged food product by the Food and Drug Administration. According to Mr. Kay, *"It meets specific standards of quality and safety from the source all the way through the finished product."* Yes, that might be true. But what Mr. Kay fails to tell you is that the packaging, i.e., plastic bottles the water is sold in contains BPA. BPA, or bisphenol A, is often found in disposable water bottles and babies' milk bottles and cups. Small amounts can dissolve into the food and drink inside these containers. The World Health Association found large quantities of BPA in bottled water. Researchers also found that 90 percent of bottled water contained microplastics. Many studies have shown that BPA mimics the actions of estrogen, binding to the same receptor in the body. BPA might be the cause of abnormal reproductive systems.

Although BPA is being phased out of plastic packaging due to public pressure and health concerns, i.e., it disrupts our hormones, research shows that the replacement might be just as dangerous. That's another illustration of unintended consequences. One replacement material is fluorene-9-bisphenol. But, research on fluorene-9-bisphenol (BHPF) has found it also attaches to the body's estrogen receptors. However, unlike BPA, BHPF does this without mimicking estrogen. Instead, PHPF blocks the estrogen receptor. This has the likelihood to create fertility problems and other issues.

Many brands of bottled water will mislead you and fool you into thinking their water is from underground springs or glaciers. It's B.S.! They are from municipal tap water. This includes two of the most popular brands, Aquafina, manufactured by PepsiCo and Dasani, produced by Coca-Cola.

Who would have imagined that plain (not to be confused with pure) water with zero calories, zero carbs, zero fat, and zero sugar could be causing you to gain weight? But unfortunately, it's true.

Research shows 80 percent of all diseases are related to our dietary behaviors and habits. This does not include the chronic illnesses correlated to our water intake, or lack thereof. Industrial chemicals are dangerous. They don't belong in our water. If you're suffering from an autoimmune disease, you should seriously test the water you're drinking. If you have a food intolerance or gastrointestinal issues like irritable bowel syndrome, the water you're drinking may be contributing to these inflammatory diseases.

For men, the water you're drinking might be the cause for low testosterone, low sperm count, or man boobs. The endocrine (hormone) damaging chemicals found in drinking water could be the culprit.

For women, are you among the 30 million Americans suffering from a thyroid issue? Is your doctor telling you this is the reason for your weight gain or inability to lose weight? It might be your water causing your weight issues.

According to the *Journal of Endocrinology*, "A very low dose of endocrine disrupting chemical exposure can have potent and irreversible effects. Research shows that the hormonal system is easily disrupted by a very minimal amount of these chemicals. They can have a negative effect on humans at very low dosages of parts per billion." *Endocrine-Disrupting Chemicals and Public Health Protection: A Statement of Principles from The Endocrine Society*, published online June 25, 2012. That means that the government agencies' statement that the amount of these endocrine disrupting chemicals found in our drinking water is so low that they're OK to consume, they are wrong. And for some of you, it means they're "dead" wrong.

So, what can you do to protect yourself from drinking contaminated water? According to Dr. David Friedman, invest in a water filter that removes these chemicals and heavy metals. But it should not be just any water filter. It needs to be a reverse osmosis system. Dr. Friedman recommends a six-phase reverse osmosis system with re-mineralization.

There are several reverse osmosis systems with seven phases and ultraviolet (UV) light bulbs on the market. Dr. Friedman does not recommend these because the UV light can heat the water to extremely hot temperatures. The high temperatures can weaken or loosen the fittings. Also, make certain the system has an NSF certification for removal of substance on the label.

David Medansky

Once you have your reverse osmosis system operating, you can use a stainless-steel bottle, a durable BPA-free bottle, or a glass bottle to bring your water with you when you're not at home.

Chapter 3

Bliss Point - Maybe It's Not Your Fault

Positive action can change every negative situation.
Darren Hardy,
New York Times best-selling author of
The Compound Effect

Most people trying to lose weight, are the uninformed being guided by the misinformed. The weight-loss industry is a misinformation machine. Why would I say this? Because Americans spend over $66 billion on weight-reduction products ranging from diet pills, herbal teas, prepared meals, and swanky gym memberships. Yet, more than 71 percent of the U.S. adult population is overweight, 41 percent of whom are clinically obese. And it's getting worse. Overconsumption is the biggest cause of weight gain.

But why is this happening?

In the movie *Good Will Hunting*, Sean Maguire (Robin Williams) tells Will (Matt Damon) "It's not your fault," over and over until Will finally understands and breaks down and cries.

Being overweight may not be your fault. Yes, we are responsible for what we put in our mouths. But, how many of you know about the "Bliss Point" or "dietary duplication?"

In this chapter, you will be warned about the dangers of the Bliss Point and processed foods much like Jacob Marley warned Ebenezer Scrooge in Charles Dicken's classic, *A Christmas Carol*. Because like Scrooge, you still have time to change.

In this chapter you will learn how most processed foods are scientifically engineered by the food industry to make them addictive and deadly. You will learn what these foods contain and why you should avoid them. At the end of this chapter some of you may feel outrage. Others might not care. But I guarantee if you pay attention, you will look at what you're eating a whole lot differently.

So, why is it so difficult for you to lose weight?

Most people fail to lose weight because:

1. It's hard to get started
2. There's no magic formula
3. It's not a quick fix
4. It's hard to sustain
5. There's no finish line
6. There's no one to be accountable to
7. Even if you know *what* to do, you might not know *how* to do it.

And, with all the information available about dieting and weight loss, who or what do you believe.

What is the Bliss Point you might be asking?

The "Bliss Point" is a term coined by Howard Moskowitz for how food manufacturers scientifically engineer our food to increase the optimization of our food tastiness and increases our cravings. Howard Moskowitz, trained in mathematics at Queens College and experimental psychology at Harvard, was hired by food manufacturers during a 30-year period starting in the 1970s to determine the perfect amount of sweetness, saltiness, texture, and richness for various products. These companies included Campbell Soups, General Foods, Kraft, and PepsiCo.

Bliss Point is used in the formulation of food products to find the perfect balance of the three main components our bodies crave – salt, sugar, and fat. It's a complex process pinpointing the exact combination of ingredients that flash our neurological pleasures zones so that we never get the "satisfaction" signal that tells us to stop eating. Like the Rolling Stones, you can't get no satisfaction.

The biggest hits — be they Coca-Cola, Doritos, or Pringles — owe their success to complex formulas that pique the taste buds enough to be alluring but don't have a distinct, overriding single flavor that tells the brain to stop eating. Simply stated, foods are engineered to be so tasty it's hard to resist them. Moskowitz describes the Bliss Point as "that sensory profile where you like the food the most." In other words, they are addicting.

Moskowitz said, "I've optimized soups, I've optimized pizzas, I've optimized salad dressings and pickles. In this field, I'm a game changer." He had no qualms about his pioneering work on discovering the Bliss Point or any of the other systems that helped food companies create the greatest amount of craving.

So, what does this mean for you?

It means food manufacturers are turning you into food junkies with the junk food they are pushing on you just like a dealer pushes illegal drugs such as meth, opioids, and heroin to junkies.

Looking back in history, this all started sometime in the 1970s when Moskowitz was commissioned to experiment and find the perfect level of sweetness for Diet Pepsi. He was instructed to find out what taste would appeal to most people.

Much to Moskowitz' surprise, the data revealed there was no bell-curve to indicate the perfect level of sweetness. What Moskowitz learned was that there was no one perfect level; only perfect levels of sweetness.

Moskowitz applied his research to his work with Prego Spaghetti Sauce. At the time, Prego had only one flavor of spaghetti sauce. Understanding there is no one perfect sauce, he developed 45 different types of spaghetti sauce for testing. Moskowitz learned that Americans fell into three groups:
- Those who liked plain spaghetti sauce,
- Those who liked chunky spaghetti sauce, and
- Those who liked spicy spaghetti sauce.

Which type of spaghetti sauce do you like?

If you like the chunky style spaghetti sauce, you can thank Dr. Moskowitz. Because before his research, no one had thought of developing a chunky-style sauce. Yet, one-third of Americans highly prefer it. The result, during the next 10 years more than $600 million in sales were generated from the extra chunky sauce line alone.

And you wonder why food manufacturers are altering our food to increase our cravings?

Vlasic's zesty pickles would not exist without Dr. Howard Moskowitz's work.

Here's another example. Cadbury Schweppes hired Moskowitz in 2004 to develop Cherry Vanilla Dr. Pepper because they wanted to expand the market for Dr. Pepper. In creating the soda, Moskowitz started with 59 variations, each slightly different than the next. He then did 3,000 taste tests around the country. The data was put through a series of math regression analyses and entered into the computer. The computer generated a bell-shaped curve to determine the perfect amount of vanilla or cherry taste to increase our craving and sell more soda.

His formulations for optimization of the amount of salt, sugar, and fat is the Bliss Point for consumer satisfaction. Food manufacturers could care less about the negative health impact it has on your dietary intake so long as they earn a profit.

Bliss Point did not stop with foods that are normally sweet. Nope. Food companies looked around grocery shelves to see what other products could be enhanced and expand their product lines. Sugar or other artificial sweeteners were added to foods that didn't use to be sweet.

Now, bread has added sugar. Some brands of yogurt can taste as sweet as ice cream. Certain brands of pasta sauce have the equivalent amount of sugar in just a half-a-cup serving as a few Oreo cookies.

In the last chapter, you learned that the average grocery store today now carries more than 50,000 products. But, in 1975 the average supermarket carried about 9,000 food products. In 1995, the average was about 35,000 products. The reason there are so many more food products is from the rapid increase of processed foods with grains and those being chemically engineered. After all, how many new fruits and vegetables have been discovered during this time?

Now you know why.

What does this mean for you?

Nutritionists say this creates an expectation that everything we eat should taste sweeter (or saltier). This is one explanation for why kids rebel against eating fresh produce. To them, it tastes bitter or sour.

As stated earlier, Moskowitz describes the Bliss Point as "that sensory profile where you like the food the most." Unfortunately, the human body has evolved to crave foods that deliver just the right amount of saltiness, richness, and sweetness. That's because your brain responds with a reward in the form of endorphins. It remembers what you did to get that reward, and makes you want to do it again.

It's an effect run by dopamine and neurotransmitters. This is the reason why you want to keep eating your junk food even though you are full. Your mind will never be satisfied. You cannot get enough - - just like a junkie on heroin. Perhaps that's why it's referred to as junk food. Because it makes you a food junkie.

Food manufacturers use combinations of sugar, fat, and salt synergistically because the combination is even more rewarding than any one alone. Their goal is to create products with two or three of these ingredients (salt, sugar, and fat) to optimize your desire to consume more and more of them and target your Bliss Point.

More Fake Foods: Fake Fat and Fake Sugar

Processed foods now contain artificial ingredients to enhance their flavor and taste. What are some of these artificial ingredients?

- Olean
- Aspartame, and
- High-fructose corn syrup.

Let's start with Olean.

What is Olean? Olean a/k/a as Olestra is one of many ingredients that resulted from Bliss Point Engineering. Proctor & Gamble created it to be a calorie and cholesterol-free fat substitute. The Food and Drug Administration (FDA) approved Olestra as a food additive in 1996, concluding that it "meets the safety standard for food additives, reasonable certainty of no harm." But, as it turned out, it is detrimental to your health. In the late 1990s, Olestra lost its popularity due to negative side effects.

Olestra was discovered accidentally by Proctor & Gamble researchers F. Mattson and R. Volpenhein in 1968 while researching fats that could be more easily digested by premature infants. A few years later, while doing more testing, Proctor & Gamble noticed olestra caused a decline in blood cholesterol levels as a side effect to replacing natural dietary fats.

Because this could be potentially very lucrative, in 1975, Proctor & Gamble filed a request with the FDA to use Olestra as a *drug* to lower cholesterol. However, the lengthy series of studies that followed all failed. Further testing and research on olestra were suspended.

1n 1984, the FDA permitted Kellogg to claim publicly that their high-fiber breakfast cereals lower the risk of cancer. This led Proctor & Gamble to start more tests on Olestra to be approved as a *food additive*. Instead of Olestra being a *drug*, P&G wanted to use Olestra as a *food additive* to replace up to 35 percent of fats in home cooking and 75 percent in commercial uses with it.

The FDA was concerned that consumers would eat more of the top of the pyramid foods because of the perception they were healthier. The FDA worried that it would cause consumers to overconsume believing that Olestra would remove negative consequences. The FDA hesitated to approve Olestra.

Proctor & Gamble, to satisfy the FDA concerns, agreed to limiting Olestra as a food additive to savory snacks that included potato chips, tortilla chips, crackers, pretzels, and similar foods. The FDA approved Olestra as a food additive in 1996 so long as it contained warning labels to warn consumers of the possible negative side effects and that vitamins were added.

Because Olestra adds no fat, calories or cholesterol to products, it is used in the preparation of otherwise high-fat foods such as potato chips, pretzels, and cookies to lower or eliminate their fat content. Since Olestra is unhealthy for you, food companies are required to put warning labels on the food products that contain it. The FDA mandated the health warning label to read,

> *This Product Contains Olestra. Olestra may cause abdominal cramping and loose stools (and leakage). Olestra inhibits the absorption of some vitamins and nutrients. Vitamins A, D, E, and K have been added.*

Proctor & Gamble argued that the label did not accurately communicate information to consumers because it was unlikely that Olestra would cause serious digestion problems. In 1996, the FDA agreed with Proctor & Gamble and stated that the label could be removed. By then, however, the damage from the negative publicity about Olestra had been done.

Undaunted, Proctor & Gamble renamed and rebranded Olestra as Olean. It's still unhealthy for you, but it is legal in the United States and it is found in many of the "fat-free" or "light" products. Olean, however, is banned in Canada, China, and the European Union (EU). You should never eat this ugly fat!

Products with Olestra/Olean are by far worse than any other fat, carb or gluten you can put into your body because this additive prevents your body from absorbing any essential vitamins and minerals. Some of the common side effects include diarrhea, cramps, leaky bowel, and gas.

Some of the brands it is found in include:
- Lays Light Potato Chips
- Pringles
- Ruffles
- Doritos

Do you snack on some of these products? Are you snacking on these products right now as you're reading this book?

When Lay's Potato Chips says, "Bet you can't eat just one." It's not a dare. It's a fact!

The FDA, for whatever reasons, still allows Olestra/Olean to be a legal food additive despite its health implications. Keep in mind that Olestra started as a drug and then became a food additive - - an artificial, scientifically engineered food additive.

Finding the Sweet Spot

Aspartame is another Bliss Point ingredient used in process foods. Aspartame is one of the most common artificial sweeteners in use today. It is sold under the brand names NutraSweet, Equal, Spoonful, and Equal-Measure.

Do you use these products?

Do you use Stevia? If so, be careful if you purchase Stevia in packets in grocery stores. Most, if not all of them, are a blend of fructose, sucrose, dextrose, and stevia or a variation thereof. Some packages will state it's a blend. Some are deceptive and won't. Be certain to read the nutrition label. In my opinion, the only place you should trust to purchase pure stevia is at Sprouts, Whole Foods, and other reputable health food stores.

Aspartame is used in many foods and beverages because it is 200 times sweeter than sugar. Food manufacturers can use less of it, thereby lowering calories in their products.

Aspartame was inadvertently discovered in 1965 by James Schlatter. Schlatter was a chemist at G.D. Searle Company testing an anti-ulcer drug.

Have you noticed the similarities between Olean and Aspartame?

Both were discovered while testing drugs. Both are artificial. That means it is not produced by nature. One of the elements for eating healthy is to eat holistic or whole foods and avoid processed foods.

Aspartame, manufactured by G.D. Searle, was approved for use in carbonated beverages in 1983. Monsanto purchased G.D. Searle in 1985.

Aspartame, manufactured by G.D. Searle, was approved for use in carbonated beverages in 1983. Monsanto, which manufactures Roundup, Agent Orange, DDT, PCB, and many insecticides, purchased G.D. Searle in 1985. Monsanto's purchase by Bayer was finalized in June 2018.

Monsanto was among the first to conduct field testing of Genetically Modified Crops. They're better known today as GMOs. GMO Foods will soon be called "Biofortified." This name change is a deliberate fraud perpetrated on you, the consumer. They did the same thing with Monosodium Glutamic Acid (MSG). MSG is a food additive that's been linked to chronic illnesses such as obesity, liver disease, high cholesterol, metabolic syndrome, neurological, brain health issues, etc. The food manufacturers changed the name of MSG to "Autolyzed Yeast" so people wouldn't know they were consuming MSG.

When the food manufacturers found the artificial sweetener aspartame caused serious health issues, they changed the name to "Amino Sweet." Don't be fooled. If Charles Manson legally changed his name to John Smith—he'd still be just as evil. Read labels.

Just be aware that the term Biofortification will have massive ramifications for the world population. In the movie *The Equalizer*, Robert McCall (Denzel Washington) tells Teri (Chloë Grace Moretz), "Change your world." Somehow, I don't believe that Biofortification food is a good change for the world. The world was a much healthier place with non-GMO foods.

Did you ever wonder why the manufacturer of pesticides, insecticides, and poison would manufacturer an ingredient used in food?

Aspartame is now found in thousands of different food products. It's commonly used as a table-top sweetener as a replacement for sugar. It is added to prepared foods and beverages that do NOT require much heating because heat breaks down aspartame.

The primary reason not to drink diet soda is that it contains Aspartame. There are 92 documented negative side effects of Aspartame. One of them is that it causes people to gain weight - *not* lose it. Aspartame affects your metabolism, so you cannot burn calories. While diet soda may contain zero calories, it will prevent you from reducing weight, and cause you to gain weight. It also inhibits or prevents your body from absorbing vitamins, minerals, and other essential nutrients. That's why it's dangerous. You are depleting your body of the proper nutrients and it goes into starvation mode, which causes weight gain. Just because Aspartame is legal, does not mean it's safe. Other reported side effects include, but are not limited to:

- Cancer
- Seizures
- Headaches
- Depression
- Attention Deficit Hyperactivity Disorder
- Weight Gain
- Birth Defects

There is controversy about this sweet deception. You will find a lot of information on the internet about aspartame. Some of these articles indicate that aspartame is safe for you. They have studies to support their claim that no health problems have been linked to aspartame. There are just as many, if not more, articles about the adverse side effects of aspartame.

This is some of what you'll learn reading up on aspartame. A 25-year study found very moderate consumption of aspartame is linked to a 65 percent higher likelihood of being overweight and a 41 percent increased likelihood of being obese. A new study shows it's toxic to your gut and sparks DNA mutations. Aspartame will ruin your health.

Many people turn to NutraSweet, Equal, or Spoonful thinking it will help them consume fewer calories, slim down and lower their risk of developing Type 2 diabetes. But researchers are now learning that's not the case. Instead, aspartame accumulates in your blood meaning your body cannot get rid of or eliminate it. This can cause even more severe damage to your blood vessels.

Yet another study has linked artificial sweeteners to impaired glucose response, suggesting they may play a role in Type 2 diabetes and can increase the risk for obesity and other related health problems.

Aspartame accounts for over 75 percent of the adverse reactions to food additives reported to the FDA. Many of these reactions are very serious.

Sweet Deception

Let's talk about the worst of the three artificial ingredients added to your food.

High-fructose corn syrup (HFCS) otherwise known as glucose-fructose, isoglucose, and glucose-fructose syrup.

How many of you know why high-fructose corn syrup has so many different names?

It's because food manufacturers know you, as a consumer, are more aware of how bad it is for you. They are attempting to disguise that their products contain HFCS by calling it something else. It's the same.

What is high-fructose corn syrup? HFCS is a sweetener *processed* from corn starch. Starches are made from long chains of linked sugars. Manufacturers break down corn starch into sweet corn syrup made of the sugar glucose. Enzymes are added to make the syrup much sweeter.

Why do manufacturers do this?

Because it's much cheaper and easier than producing sucrose, which is ordinary table sugar. The ratio of fructose to glucose is nearly the same as HFCS to table sugar. Both have 4 calories per gram.

Studies show that animals, such as chickens, that eat a high-fructose corn syrup diet gain more weight than those that don't. How many of you are starting to understand that because many chicken breeders are feeding their birds diets high in HFCS chickens are getting bigger and bigger? A plumper bird returns a higher price. It's all about the profit margins. Your health be damned.

HFCS was first marketed in the early 1970s by the *Clinton Corn Processing Company* of Clinton, Iowa. It is composed of 76 percent carbohydrates and 24 percent water. It contains no fat, no protein, and no essential nutrients. One tablespoon has 53 calories.

HFCS is found in sodas, desserts, some breakfast cereals, and elsewhere. It is linked to obesity, diabetes, and even some forms of cancer.

There is a debate as to whether HFCS is unhealthy for you. You can find studies done to support that it's *not* harmful. The question I'll pose to you is if HFCS is not harmful to your health or doesn't have negative side effects, then why go through the trouble of calling it by different names on the Nutrition Facts label?

Avoid anything ending in "OSE." That includes dextrose, sucrose, glucose, fructose, and isoglucose. You get the idea.

What's in Your Sandwich?

A sandwich with a few slices of deli meat is a cheap and quick brown-bag lunch. How many of you make sandwiches to take to work?

Unfortunately, sandwiches made with deli meat or processed meats have been linked to increased risk of cancer, diabetes, and heart disease.

How many of you are wondering what deli meats or processed meats actually are?

Ham, bacon, pastrami, salami, and bologna are *processed meats*. So are sausages, hot dogs, bratwursts, and frankfurters.

In 2007, a review of 7,000 studies found convincing evidence that high intakes of processed meat increased the risk of colorectal cancer.

It was thought that chronic obstructive pulmonary disease (COPD) was primarily caused by cigarette smoking. COPD was the third most common cause of death worldwide in 2010. But up to one-third of patients who contracted COPD had never smoked. This suggested that other factors were involved. Until recently, little attention had been paid to these other factors, such as diet.

An article published in the *European Respiratory Journal*, Volume 43, Issue 4 published on March 31, 2014, found that a steady diet of processed meats (bacon, gammon, ham, corned beef, spam, and luncheon meat, sausage, meat pies, etc.) was linked with worse lung function, in both males and females. Further, health professionals determined that cured meat consumption was directly related to newly diagnosed COPD cases. And another study in Spain of patients with COPD showed that everyday consumption of cured deli meats exacerbated COPD symptoms and condition.

In 2015, the World Health Organization classified processed meats as "carcinogenic to humans" and red meat as "probably carcinogenic." Red meat is any meat from a mammal (for example beef, veal, pork, goat, lamb, and bison).

Another recent study found that people who ate more than 160 grams of processed meat (160 grams of processed meat is equivalent to two large Italian sausages or three slices of deli ham and three small hot dogs) each day – versus less than 20 grams – were 44 percent more likely to die early from cardiovascular disease or cancer.

What makes processed meat so unhealthy? For starters, it's a source of saturated fat, the type that raises blood cholesterol. It's also very high in sodium. Four strips of cooked bacon, for example, packs 800 milligrams, more than half a day's worth. And, it has high amounts of nitrates and nitrites.

Sodium nitrates and sodium nitrites are salt compounds that naturally occur in the soil and are in many fruits and vegetables, such as celery, leafy greens, and cabbage. In fact, most of the nitrates we eat come from vegetables and drinking water. When nitrates contact with saliva in the mouth, they convert to nitrites.

Sodium nitrate is added to cold cuts for preservation and to inhibit bacteria growth. Nitrate is converted to sodium nitrite when it connects with bacteria in the meat. Most manufacturers now directly add nitrite to the meat. Nitrates and nitrites themselves do not cause cancer, but there is a concern that they may produce carcinogenic compounds in the body or during processing or cooking.

Frances Largeman-Roth, R.D.N., a nutrition expert and author of Eating in Color, says, "We know that when nitrites combine with the amines in meat, they create nitrosamines, which some studies have found to be carcinogenic."

Because consumers are wary, some manufacturers now cure meats with celery powder since celery is naturally high in nitrate. These meats are labeled "uncured" and "celery powder" is in the ingredients list instead of "sodium nitrite."

Cooking meat at high temperatures forms heterocyclic amines, compounds that have been linked to cancer in animals and colorectal polyps in people.

Am I suggesting you eliminate eating processed meats all together? No, of course not! I'll still enjoy bacon with my eggs on occasion or a hot dog. But, it's not part of my normal eating routine. I enjoy them, but rarely, such as at a baseball game or at a friend's BBQ.

How many of you are wondering what are some healthier alternatives?

Healthier alternatives for sandwiches and wraps include tuna, salmon, hummus and veggies, or fresh, cooked poultry. When you're baking or grilling chicken, cook extra for lunches during the week.

Or, roast a whole fresh turkey breast on Sunday to slice up for sandwiches and salads during the week.

Google or watch a YouTube video on how to make a Mediterranean wrap. Remember, it's more than just the meat. It's about the bread, cheese, mayo, and other condiments that people, like maybe yourself, add to their sandwiches. When you add up all the sodium, fats, sugars, and nitrates from the ingredients in a sub sandwich, club sandwich, or "specialty" sandwich at your favorite restaurant - Yikes.

Let's talk about bread, the foundation of every sandwich. White flour, which is used to make white bread, is the absolute worst, since the bleaching process that it undergoes strips away all the nutrients. Consuming white bread can cause a spike in blood sugar, weight gain, and inflammation.

Whole-grain bread, not to be confused with multi-grain, is a much better choice. It's loaded with fiber, healthy plant-based protein, vitamins, minerals and a variety of phytochemicals that help to improve digestion, reduce inflammation, and lower cholesterol. Whole-grain bread also contains lactic acid, which promotes the growth of good bacteria in the intestines. Rye bread is another healthy option. Research published in the "Nutritional Journal" shows that rye bread can help decrease hunger for up to eight hours.

In his blog, Dr. David Freidman, author of the international award-winning, number one best-selling book, *Food Sanity*, ranked sandwiches from healthiest to unhealthiest. According to Dr. Friedman, the turkey sandwich (roasted turkey, not processed) is the healthiest because it contains less fat than most other meats and it's rich in protein and potassium. Turkey also contains tryptophan, which helps support healthy levels of serotonin, our good mood chemical. It's best to go with pasture-raised turkey if possible because it provides more heart-healthy omega-3 fatty acids than factory-farmed turkey.

Adding cheese to your lean turkey sandwich, however, can add a lot of fat and calories. For example, two slices of cheddar contain a whopping 226 calories and 18 grams of fat — not to mention, most cheese is loaded with sodium. Instead of cheese, add some healthy lettuce, tomatoes, and onions, and you have a heart-healthy sandwich. Some of the other sandwiches discussed by Dr. Friedman included:

Egg Salad. A common misconception is that eggs contribute to high cholesterol and heart disease. The truth is, eggs are a nutritional super food. Eggs contain lecithin which helps lower cholesterol levels and protects against heart disease. When it comes to egg salad, hold the mayo. Just two tablespoons pack on 188 calories and 20 grams of fat.

Tuna makes for a great sandwich. It provides 80 percent of our daily recommended amount of selenium which research shows may help prevent cancer. It's also high in omega-3 fatty acids, which is important for heart health and brain function. Three ounces of canned tuna only contains 108 calories. Add some chopped celery to your tuna salad for added fiber. It also helps support a healthy immune system. Or, eat it without the bread.

Peanut Butter and Jelly Sandwiches. Peanut butter and jelly sandwiches can be quite healthy at any age. Peanut butter is a great source of protein, B vitamins, iron, and zinc. Peanut butter is also a good choice for healthy unsaturated fat and will keep you full for hours. However, avoid peanut butter with a bunch of added oils or sugar. There should only be two ingredients: peanuts and salt. If you have an allergy to peanuts, use almond or cashew butter.

For a healthier PBJ, use jam instead of jelly. Jam won't spike your blood sugar as much as jelly because it contains the whole fruit, which helps to buffer the glycemic load (how quickly sugar enters your bloodstream.) If you're not fond of jam, use honey. Raw honey is loaded with vitamins, enzymes, and powerful antioxidants.

The **Bacon, Lettuce, and Tomato (BLT)** sandwich or club sandwich. Americans love bacon. The popular keto diet advocates consuming bacon and many people are doing that daily. However, there's no research showing that bacon is healthy — in fact, evidence shows quite the opposite. *The American Institute for Cancer Research* performed one of the most in-depth studies to date. Their conclusion: "Processed meat should be avoided for life."

Traditional Grilled Cheese Sandwich made with American cheese. Unfortunately, two slices contain 220 calories (90 of them from fat,) 12 grams of saturated fat and 360 mg of sodium.

Ham and Cheese. Ham isn't the healthiest meat option because it falls into the "processed meat" category. Research published in *PLOS Medicine* found that eating ham may increase your risk for colon and lung cancer. Ham is also high in sodium. An average sized ham sandwich contains 1000 milligrams of sodium.

The **Meatball Marinara Sub** is extremely unhealthy and fattening. A Subway 12-inch meatball marinara sub has 1,160 calories! But you can still eat at Subway in a healthy manner. As an alternative to their fresh baked bread, have a flatbread. For me, I keep it simple. A 6-inch tuna on whole wheat flatbread, *no* cheese, with spinach, cucumber, green pepper, and avocado if they have it. That's it. Very simple and healthy.

According to Dr. Friedman, the **Philadelphia Cheesesteak** ranks as his pick for the most-unhealthy sandwich. It's high in calories and loaded with grease, salt, and fat. 12-inch cheesesteak with provolone, peppers, onions, and mushrooms packs a whopping 1,278 calories and 27.5 grams of saturated fat — that's not including the greasy fries that often come with it (add another 364 calories). A Philly cheesesteak also contains 1,480 milligrams of salt.

If you're serious about shedding your unwanted pounds and getting rid of that extra weight, simply avoid eating a sandwich.

Next time you're at a restaurant check out the menu to see what they state are the calories for each dish. You might be shocked. And, that's just the calories. Most places will not provide you with how much sugar, salt, or fat is in an item being served.

If you look at the packaging of processed foods in the grocery store, it will tell you about the low sodium, low fat, low calories and so forth. But what they might not tell you, is the number of carbohydrates or other information that is unhealthy because it's such a large quantity. For example, the front of some spaghetti boxes might state, "0 cholesterol, 0 sodium, low fat or no fat, 0 sugar." And many of you might be thinking "that sounds good." Yes, it does. What they don't tout or promote is it has 42g of carbohydrates per serving. That's more than a typical ice cream sandwich, Hagen Daaz, or Dove ice cream bar. Those have between 26g and 34 grams of carbohydrates. If you're reducing weight, you need to avoid the spaghetti.

Keep in mind, it's more than just calories in and calories out if you're attempting to reduce weight in a healthy manner that's sustainable. Achieving and maintaining a healthy weight is about choices. We all have choices. Why wait until you're in a health crisis if it can be avoided?

The American Heart Association recommends eating no more than 2,300 mg of sodium per day (for some groups even less), but we're consuming much more. Kids in the U.S. eat an average of 3,279 mg of sodium per day. Adults average more than 3,400 mg/day.

With cold cuts, the sodium adds up quickly given that just one ounce of deli turkey can have more than 500 mg of sodium. A slice of cheese has 150 mg. Each slice of bread has 140 mg. One sandwich may be close to 1,000 mg of sodium, not including any extra condiments like mustard or mayo. That's almost half of our daily requirement in one part of a meal.

Since the mid-1980s medical research has known that 80 percent of the three leading causes of premature death are, 1) overconsumption of processed food, 2) smoking tobacco, and 3) inactivity. Dr. David L. Katz refers to these as the three "F's".

Food – over eating processed foods

Fingers – used for smoking

Feet – lack of walking, running or other physical activity

Bliss Point used to create processed foods has caused many of today's chronic diseases. Chronic diseases take life from years and years from life. Dr. Katz says, "I'm all about adding life to years and years to life."

How many of you remember that obesity now causes more deaths than smoking?

And, four out of every ten U.S. adults are clinically obese.

What does that mean for you?

It means that you're more likely to die from overeating than from smoking. In society today, it's no longer health care – it's disease care. According to the 2017 Bloomberg Global Health Index, the United States ranks 34th in the world for health. The U.S. ranking of 34 out of 163 countries who met the criteria to be evaluated was negatively impacted because of the prevalence of overweight people.

Imagine making some small adjustments to your daily eating routines that you do consistently over a long period of time to give you noticeable results, such as a smaller waistline, having more energy, being able to spend more time with the kids or grand-kids and being physically active with them, and lowering your risk for expensive medical ailments, even death.

Hydrogenated Oil

Hydrogenated oils are vegetable oils whose chemical structure has been altered to prevent rancidity in foods, which increases shelf life and saves money for food manufacturers. The process of hydrogenation involves the addition of hydrogen atoms to the oil's available double bonds. As the level of hydrogenation increases, the level of saturated fat increases and the level of unsaturated fat decreases.

The hydrogenation process converts what are known as "cis" double bonds to "trans" double bonds. During this manufactured partially hydrogenated processing, a type of fat called trans fat is created. Food manufacturers like hydrogenation because it has the technical advantage of making foods solid or partially solid at room temperature.

Food companies prefer using hydrogenated oil because it does extend the shelf life of products and save costs. This comes at a cost. Trans fats raise total blood cholesterol levels and LDL and increase your risk for heart disease. There are two types of trans fats found in food: 1) naturally occurring and 2) artificial, where they add hydrogen to the liquid oil (partially hydrogenated oil). In other words, hydrogenated oil is another processed food used in the preparation of what you're being given to eat.

These partially hydrogenated oils block the production of chemicals that combat inflammation and benefit the hormonal and nervous systems, while at the same time allowing chemicals that increase inflammation. This means that trans fats promote inflammation and negatively impact cholesterol levels.

The Harvard School of Public Health notes that trans fats promote immune system over-activity and inflammation and are linked to heart disease, stroke, and diabetes, among other chronic diseases. One 2006 article published in the *New England Journal of Medicine* noted that at that time the average American consumed nearly 5 grams of trans fat per day -- an amount that increases the risk for heart disease by approximately 25 percent.

The artificial trans fats are:

- Easy to use
- Inexpensive to produce – it's cheap. More profits for the food providers.
- Used to increase stability and extend the shelf life of products.
- Used to enhance the texture of food.
- Used by many restaurants and fast food outlets to deep fry foods because trans fat can be used many times in a commercial fryer.

On the other hand, *fully* hydrogenated oil contains very little trans fats and doesn't have the same health risks as trans fats. Because partially hydrogenated oil contains trans fats, it's best to avoid any food that contains it. Partially hydrogenated oil is found in:

- Margarine
- Microwave popcorn
- Cakes, pies, and cookies
- Doughnuts
- Vegetable shortening
- Packaged snacks
- Baked foods, especially premade versions
- Ready-to-use-dough (Thank you Pillsbury Doughboy)
- Fried foods (Onion rings, French fries, fried zucchini)
- Coffee creamers, both dairy and non-dairy

Partially hydrogenated oil isn't always easy to spot, but there are ways to spot it and avoid it.

Some food labels claim they have no trans fats, but partially hydrogenated oil may be listed as one of the ingredients. It's important to read both the Nutrition Facts label and the ingredients list.

Food preservation goes hand in hand with packaged foods – longer shelf life. Decrease or eliminate your dependency on packaged foods. For example, cook your own brown rice (avoid white rice) or potatoes from scratch instead of purchasing the boxed versions. Yes, it's quicker and more convenient to prepare the boxed version. But this is where you get to choose what you want to put into your body.

Consider baking or broiling your foods rather than frying them. Use heart-healthy oils such as safflower, olive, or avocado oil.

I'm amazed at how many people are concerned about air pollution and water pollution but have no qualms about polluting their own bodies.

Consider preparing your own snacks. Some ideas for healthy, great tasting snacks include:

- Raw unsalted nuts such as walnuts, pecans, and almonds
- Carrot sticks
- Celery
- Apples
- Berries such as blueberries, strawberries, raspberries, and blackberries
- Raw cheese (avoid processed pasteurized cheese if possible)
- Plain Greek yogurt without the added fruit. It's best to add your own berries or fruit

Let's Discuss Dietary Duplication

Dietary duplication is a term coined by an acquaintance of mine, John Canida. It means you eat like your parents because that is how you were raised. We all like certain foods more than others because of what our parents fed us.

If you think you are overweight because of genetics, most likely you are wrong. Think back to how you were raised and what your parents served you for meals. Do you have a favorite dish prepared by your mother, father, or grandparent? Probably most, if not everyone does. Think of your eating patterns and how you prepare your foods.

Did you eat dinner at the kitchen or dining room table as a family? Or, did you go through the drive-thru often? Perhaps your parents ordered pizza to be delivered. Or, maybe they picked one up on the way home.

Maybe you ate your dinner while watching TV. Or ate while working in front of your computer? Perchance you had your meal while doing homework.

Can you remember your parents being rushed or too tired to cook and it was easier for them to order a pizza, pick up a bucket of KFC, or microwave your dinner?

These are the habits you learned while growing up. For many of you, it's normal.

You will learn in future chapters how to make small adjustments to change and improve your eating behaviors so that they become new habits that will help you achieve a healthier weight and more importantly, maintain it. Yes, you can have a transformation for a healthier lifestyle.

You will learn not only *what* to do, but *how* to do it in future lessons. The choice is yours. In Chapter One you'll recall we agreed that nothing about your eating habits will change unless you do something different. My warning to you is to avoid any food that has a TV commercial. At the very least, reduce how much of the food advertised on television you eat.

Let's review what you can start doing now:

- Drink more pure water. More than 70 percent of the U.S. population suffers from dehydration. When we are thirsty, we tend to eat incorrectly, thinking we are hungry.
- Avoid sodas and diet sodas
- Reduce or eliminate your alcohol consumption
- If possible, avoid eating after 7:00 p.m.
- Use a salad plate instead of a dinner plate
- Eat slower
- Get adequate sleep

Here's a tip you can use. If you have a craving for food you know you shouldn't indulge in, brush your teeth. Research has shown that people with a clean mouth are less likely to snack or eat junk food.

At this time, many of you might be wondering what is the best diet to lose weight quickly? The truth about healthy and sustainable weight reduction, to some extent, is in plain sight. Rather like the infamous elephant in the room.

As you will recall, Dr. David L. Katz, author of several books, including his most recent, *The Truth About Food, Why Pandas Eat Bamboo and People Get Bamboozled* gives a simple formula:

- Eat holistic (whole) foods
- Mostly plants
- Not too much
- Avoid processed foods, and
- Drink lots of pure water

When we talk about the fractured parts of proper nutrition and diet, it's a truth some of you might feel you already know. Others might be confused by it. But, according to Dr. Katz, there's the one thing, we can all learn from looking at the elephant in the room. It's based on the poem *Blind Men and the Elephant* – by John Godfrey Saxe. Below is John Godfrey Saxe's (1816-1887) version of: Blind Men and the Elephant.

Blind Men and the Elephant

It was six men of Indostan,
To learning much inclined,
Who went to see the Elephant
(Though all of them were blind),
That each by observation
Might satisfy his mind.

The *First* approach'd the Elephant,
And happening to fall
Against his broad and sturdy side,

At once began to bawl:
"God bless me! but the Elephant
Is very like a wall!"

The *Second*, feeling of the tusk,
Cried, -"Ho! what have we here
So very round and smooth and sharp?
To me 'tis mighty clear,
This wonder of an Elephant
Is very like a spear!"

The *Third* approach'd the animal,
And happening to take
The squirming trunk within his hands,
Thus boldly up and spake:
"I see," -quoth he- "the Elephant
Is very like a snake!"

The *Fourth* reached out an eager hand
And felt about the knee.
"What most this wondrous beast is like
Is mighty plain," -quoth he, -
"Tis clear enough the Elephant
Is very like a tree!"

The *Fifth*, who chanced to touch the ear,
Said- "E'en the blindest man
Can tell what this resembles most;
Deny the fact who can,
This marvel of an Elephant
Is very like a fan!"

The *Sixth* no sooner had begun
About the beast to grope,
Then, seizing on the swinging tail
That fell within his scope,

"I see," -quoth he, -"the Elephant
Is very like a rope!"

And so, these men of Indostan
Disputed loud and long,
Each in his own opinion
Exceeding stiff and strong,
Though each was partly in the right,
And all were in the wrong!

MORAL,
So, oft in theologic wars
The disputants, I ween,
Rail on in utter ignorance
Of what each other mean;
And prate about an Elephant
Not one of them has seen!

When you ask which one is "the best-diet," be it the Keto Diet, Mediterranean Diet, Paleo Diet, South Beach, Atkins, Nutrisystem, Weight Watchers, Medifast, Jenny Craig, The Biggest Loser Diet, or others touted by medical doctors and celebrities, keep in mind the poem about the elephant and the six blind men. For each has its good features and each has its bad features. But none gives a balanced approach for a lifestyle transformation. Diets are only a momentary fix. They do not address the underlying issues. Diets are temporary, extreme, and unsustainable.

Besides, who wants to remain on a diet for the rest of their life? Think in terms of making a lifestyle change.

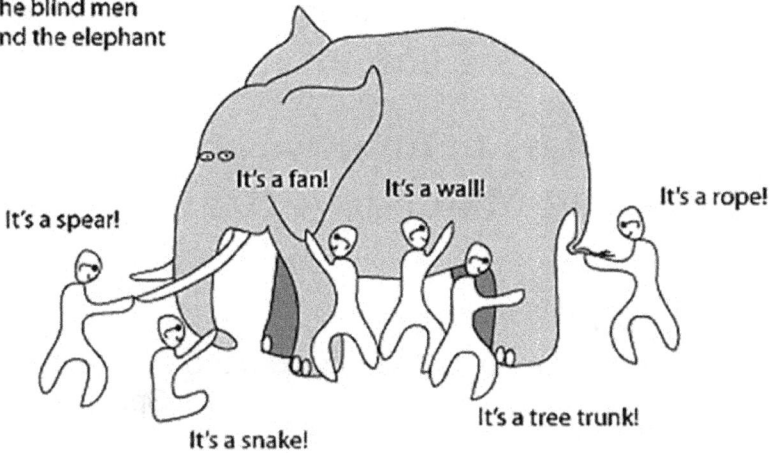

The blind men and the elephant

It's a fan!
It's a wall!
It's a rope!
It's a spear!
It's a snake!
It's a tree trunk!

As you will recall, in Chapter One I asked that you each keep an open mind. The six blind men and the elephant is one reason why.

In the next chapter, we will discuss 10 eating behaviors you can change and improve to help you on your weight-loss journey. In future chapters and throughout this book we will discuss the mindset of healthy weight-loss and the emotional, mental, and psychological aspects of it. Darren Hardy said, "What you expect is what you manifest, what you create. Have positive expectancy." Therefore, envision your weight-reduction journey going well.

Chapter 4

Ten Behaviors to Improve and Change to Achieve and Maintain A Healthy Weight

A man too busy to take care of his health is like a
mechanic too busy to take care of his tools.
Spanish Proverb

Abraham Lincoln said, "Live a good life. And in the end, it's not the years in a life, but it's the life in the years." Translation: It's about the quality of your life, not just how long you live.

In the past, did you jump right into dieting and losing weight without any planning or thought like so many others? Then what happens? You find yourself overwhelmed and stressed because you have no plan to follow. The result is poor performance and failure. People decide they want to lose weight, choose a diet without much research or planning, then fail because they get distracted, make exceptions, and lose focus.

In this chapter, you'll learn to create a weekly plan, a course of action. You will also learn ten eating behaviors to focus on changing and improving. Do them one at a time. Focus on that single behavior for an entire day, then a week, then a month.

Once you have mastered that behavior so that it becomes a habit, move on to the next behavior to implement change and improvement. Once you mastered the new behavior to modify and improve upon for an entire month, repeat the process with different behaviors.

Keep that discipline up for 90 days and you will find you have some new behaviors – healthy habits. But that's just the beginning. You are changing your lifestyle, and that is, quite frankly, harder than dieting. Within six months to a year, your food and beverage eating habits will be improved. And you should have noticeable weight-reduction results.

Don't overwhelm yourself with too many rules and expectations. Focus on one eating behavior to improve and master each month. The trick is to keep it up.

Start Today!

Commit to doing this long-term, because a behavior needs to be repeated, consistently, and long enough to form a habit. A habit is something you do without thinking about it.

The 10 eating behaviors to change and improve are:

1. Drink more pure water
2. Avoid processed foods
3. Eat whole or holistic foods
4. Read and understand nutrition labels
5. Reduce portion sizes
6. Eat slower
7. Reduce or avoid alcoholic beverages
8. Watch your thoughts, watch your words -they have impact
9. Stop eating after 7:00 p.m.
10. Get adequate sleep

Knowing *what* to do is a start. In this chapter, you'll also learn how to improve and change your eating for each behavior mentioned.

But before we get into the specifics, you need to get the background behind this philosophy.

Changing and improving daily habits is a key component of your weight-reduction success and healthy weight management. This is important. You don't have to modify all your bad habits at one time to significantly improve your life. Darren Hardy said, "The moment you choose not to pay the price of success is the moment you choose to suffer the consequences of failure, which is the worst kind of suffering."

With respect to weight loss, the greatest battle we face is prioritizing our eating habits and behaviors. We all start with grand intentions to lose weight, but then we are overcome by the irresistible call of unhealthy foods and beverages. The instant gratification and comfort from these processed foods and artificially sweetened beverages overwhelms our senses and are hard to resist. They beckon us to choose them over healthier, nourishing foods and beverages.

The problem is how to determine fact from fiction, truth from the myths, and the correct data from the fabricated, with the continuous swirling flow of "diet" information. Have you experienced the emotional anguish of having set your weight-reduction intentions for the week only to see them get derailed and sidetracked? Have you felt frustrated and regretful at the end of the week? I know how it feels because that's exactly how I felt.

Now, imagine starting each week with unwavering confidence knowing exactly what to focus on and how to handle adverse situations, challenges, or obstacles toward achieving a healthy and sustainable weight. You'll have a plan.

Achieving your healthy and sustainable weight is possible without having to order special foods, follow restrictive recipes, follow an exercise program, take drugs, undergo surgeries, or calculate food exchanges. How?

It's okay to jump into a diet, but don't try to do all the behavior changes at once. By making small improvements to your eating habits and behaviors consistently over a long period of time, one year; you will see noticeable results. "One year!" you exclaim. "But..." Remember, I told you this is not a diet. You are changing your behaviors and your lifestyle.

If you lost just two, three or four pounds each month for 12 consecutive months, you'd weigh 24 to 48 pounds less within one year. Diets are a temporary fix, usually extreme and unsustainable. Improving and changing your food and beverage choices and habits is a permanent lifestyle change that will provide lifetime benefits.

The approach you will learn in this lesson is based on the Keystone Habit discussed by Charles Duhigg in his book, *The Power of Habit*, whereby changing one key habit can change your entire life. A keystone habit is more important than others because they lead to the development of other habits. While they don't necessarily create a direct cause-and-effect relationship, they start a chain effect that produces other positive outcomes.

Charles Duhigg told the story how Paul O'Neill changed one Keystone Habit to transform the American Aluminum Company of America, also known as ALCOA, a corporation that manufactures everything from the foil that wraps Hershey's Kisses and the metal in Coca Cola cans to the bolts that hold satellites together, into an extremely profitable organization and a mainstay of safety.

According to Duhigg, after Paul O'Neill became the new CEO of ALCOA, he spoke with Wall Street Investors and stock analysts on a blustery day in October 1987. A few minutes before noon, O'Neill took the stage and said, "I want to talk to you about worker safety. Every year, numerous ALCOA workers are injured so badly that they miss a day of work. I intend to make ALCOA the safest company in America. I intend to go for zero injuries."

The audience was confused. Usually, a new CEO talks about profit margins, new markets, and collaboration. But O'Neill said nothing about profits. He didn't mention any usual business buzzwords.

Eventually, a person in the audience asked about inventories in the aerospace division. Another asked about the company's capital ratio. O'Neill responded, "I'm not certain you heard me. If you want to understand how ALCOA is doing, you need to look at our workplace safety figures. Profits do not matter as much as safety."

When the presentation ended, the investors and analyst bolted out the doors. One investor dashed to the lobby to find the nearest payphone. He called 20 of his largest clients and told them, "There's a crazy hippie in charge who is going to kill the company." He strongly suggested and advised them to sell ALCOA's stock without delay.

Later, that same adviser admitted it was the worst piece of advice he gave in his entire career. Within a year of O'Neill's speech, ALCOA profits soared to a record high. By the time O'Neill left ALCOA in 2000 to become Treasury Secretary, ALCOA's annual net income was five times larger than before he arrived.

So how did O'Neill transform ALCOA, a large, dull, and dangerous company to work for into an extremely profitable organization and one of the safest companies to work? By attacking one area of interest, ALCOA's concern for safety – a Keystone Habit. That single change to improve safety rippled throughout the entire organization.

O'Neill said, "I knew I had to transform ALCOA. But you can't order people to change."

This same concept applies to weight reduction. We all know what to do, we just don't do it. No one can order or command you to change your eating habits and behaviors. Again, this is the simple formula to achieving a healthy weight and maintaining it:

- Eat holistic (whole) foods
- Mostly plants,
- Not too much,
- Avoid processed foods, and
- Drink lots of pure water.

I added one more element to Dr. Katz's formula: Get adequate sleep.

As to forcing people to comply with directions, O'Neill said, "That's not how the brain works. So, I decided I was going to start by focusing on one thing. If I could start disrupting the habits around one thing, it would spread throughout the entire company." This can work for you in your personal life and weight-reduction journey. Just pick one Keystone Habit or one key behavior to change. Focus on improving one thing. It could be one aspect of the food or beverages you eat or drink or one behavior you do while eating a meal. Just pick one to start.

In 2009, a group of researchers funded by the National Institute of Health published a study of a different approach to weight loss. They asked 1,600 participants to write down everything they ate for at least one day per week. After six months, those who kept a food log lost twice as much weight as those who didn't. The researchers learned that many participants started looking at their entries and finding patterns they didn't know existed. They started different behaviors the researchers had not suggested. Some noticed they seemed to snack at 10 a.m. so they started keeping an apple or banana in their desks for a midmorning snack. Others started using their journals to plan future menus, and at dinner, they ate healthier rather than fast food or junk food in the fridge. But this Keystone Habit – food journaling- created a structure that helped the participants improve other habits. We'll discuss more about food journals in Chapter Six.

David J. Schwartz, Ph.D., author of *The Magic of Thinking Big*, said, "When you believe, your mind finds ways to do!" If you believe it's the smallest changes to your eating habits and lifestyle done consistently over time (more than one year) that can make the biggest difference to successfully reduce weight and keep it off, you'll succeed.

Darren Hardy provided the inspiration for this blueprint to change and improve your eating behaviors to achieve your weight reduction goals with weekly planning in his *Sunday Planning System.* He suggested not to get caught up into the complete makeover or the life renovation idea because it will end up being too much, triggering a collapse in discipline.

Hardy explained that radically making a change or going to an extreme will bring the entire weight-loss process down like a house of cards. Darren Hardy, like Charles Duhigg, trusts that if you disrupt the habit of doing one thing it will spread throughout your entire lifestyle.

Each Sunday plan your week. Plan your meals. Plan how you will handle certain situations that may pose a challenge or obstacle to sticking to your new eating habits.

Set the behavior you want to improve for the week. Focus on one or two behaviors to improve upon each week.

When you focus on changing and improving one key habit, you will notice it will have a ripple effect on your body, mind, and spirit and positively affect almost every other aspect of your life. People fail to reduce weight in a healthy and sustainable manner because they lose focus, make exceptions, and get side-tracked. Each year, people make resolutions to lose weight. Eighty percent of those will fail within the first few weeks. They are not committed to reducing weight. Commitment, according to Darren Hardy is defined as,

"Doing the thing you said you were going to do long after the mood you said it has left you."

Before we get into HOW to change and improve your daily eating routines, I'd like to offer you a daily ritual to start each day. It is optional. You only need to do it if you choose to do so. Read the words below, out loud, to start each new day.

- I begin the day expecting amazing things.
- I begin the day being grateful for what I have and what I will receive.
- I begin the day open to receiving new ideas, new information, and new connections.
- I begin the day letting go of what's not serving me. Some refer to this as "bless and release."
- I begin the day being a positive influence on others.
- "I am whole, perfect, strong, powerful, loving, harmonious,[grateful, healthy] and happy." Charles Haanel
- Napoleon Hill began his day reciting, "O Divine Providence, I ask not for more riches, but more wisdom with which to make wiser use of the riches you gave me at birth, consisting in the power to control and direct my own mind to whatever ends I desire."

Behavior #1: Drink More Pure Water

If you drink soda or diet soda, switch to drinking pure water. If you don't like water, figure out a way to enhance the taste by adding lemon, orange, watermelon, cucumber, pineapple, or other fruits and berries to give it a delicious, thirst quenching flavor. Have you been on vacation to a tropical place such as the Caribbean or South Pacific? Did you ever notice that the water served in the hotel or resort lobby is enhanced with various fruits and berries?

How about at those expensive resorts where they serve water flavored with fresh cucumber orange, lemon, or other fruits and berries. Does it make you feel special?

Imagine feeling special every day by enjoying a fresh glass of delicious water that is not artificially flavored.

Do you believe you drink enough water each day?

If you are honest, you would admit that you're not.

How do I know this? Because, in 2013, CBS reported that up to 75 percent of the American population suffered from a chronic state of dehydration. What this means for you is if you are at a social gathering with 10 others, less than three of you are properly hydrated. The other seven are suffering from chronic dehydration.

Our bodies are composed of 60 percent water. Our muscles are comprised of 75 percent water. Our brains contain 85 percent water. Are you starting to understand the importance of drinking more pure water each day?

Americans buy more soda than water. Let me repeat that. Americans purchase more soda than water. Proper hydration is vital to achieving and maintaining good health. So, why do we continue to ignore this one simple change and improvement that can be made to our daily eating behaviors?

Maybe some of you know the answer. I'll admit I don't. Perhaps it's because you're taking your good health for granted because we don't realize the damage being done to our bodies gradually until we are confronted with a chronic illness, heart attack, stroke, or some form of cancer.

Think about this for a few minutes, our bodies are comprised of approximately 60 percent water. Not soda. Water. Yet, Americans purchase more soda and drink more soda than water.

Often, if you think you're hungry, most likely you are thirsty. Instead of reaching for an unhealthy snack or a quick meal at the drive-thru window, drink a glass of water. Grace Webb, Assistant Director for Clinical Nutrition at New York Hospital said, "People just think that when they start to get a little weak or they have a headache, they need to eat something, but most often they need to drink." I'd add, drink pure water, not a soda or diet soda.

If possible, drink your water at room temperature without ice. It's easier to gulp a glass of water at room temperature water than ice cold water.

Water is necessary for the body to digest and absorb vitamins and nutrients. It also detoxifies the liver and kidneys and carries waste away. Over time, failure to drink enough water can contribute to a wide array of medical complications, from fatigue, joint pain, and weight gain to headaches, ulcers, high blood pressure, and kidney disease.

Are you ready to drink more water each day? We shall see.

Behavior #2: Avoid Processed Foods

This was discussed at length in the previous chapter. But, as a quick refresher,

- Avoid and forego consuming deli meats.
- Avoid and forego ingesting chips, pretzels, cookies, crackers, etc.
- Avoid canned soups or frozen meals that need to be microwaved.

Behavior #3: Eat Holistic (Whole) Foods

In today's fast-paced, high-demand world, our culture has focused on convenience, and that includes how we eat. When we are hungry, it's much easier to go to the drive-thru, open a can, unwrap a package or pop a lid than it is to prepare a fresh meal. But according to holistic nutritionists, the cost of convenience has a dramatic impact on your health. With the epidemic rise of obesity and diabetes, the link to your health and what you eat has taken center stage. Many of you might be looking for a way not only to feed your bodies but heal yourself as well.

What are holistic foods? Holistic food is eating healthy food as close to its natural state as possible for optimum health and wellbeing. Hallmarks of holistic foods include unrefined, unprocessed, organic, and locally grown whole foods. Holistic or whole foods are foods that have been grown and nourished from the earth rather than manufactured and sold in a package. The significance between these two kinds of foods lies in the difference in nutrient content. Fruits, vegetables, legumes, beans, nuts, seeds, and whole grains are a rich source of the vitamins and minerals that our bodies require.

Although processed foods may be enriched or enhanced with vitamins and minerals, they are rarely in the forms most bioavailable to our bodies. When you eat food that is vibrant and alive, you invite that vitality into your own body. Hippocrates said, "Let food be thy

medicine and medicine be thy food." By choosing to eat more whole or holistic foods, you may experience health benefits, such as:
- Weight loss
- Increased energy levels
- Improved mood
- Better sleep
- Improved skin tone and texture
- Strengthened immune system
- Balanced blood sugar levels
- Reduced cholesterol and blood pressure levels
- Improved digestion and relief from constipation

Additionally, you may lower your risk for chronic illnesses that can be prevented or improved through diet, such as:
- Type 2 diabetes
- Arthritis
- Heart disease
- High blood pressure
- Cancer
- Colitis
- Gout

Eating whole, raw foods is the simplest form to provide your body with proper nourishment. For a healthy snack, eat an apple, banana, carrot, celery, grapes, melon, avocado, or your favorite fruit or vegetable the way nature intended – raw and unprocessed.

Another thing you can do is eliminate white flour or white rice because the white varieties are stripped of most of their nutrition and fiber. Other suggestions to eat whole foods and accomplish an eating behavior improvement and change:
- Eat cherries and nuts (unsalted/raw) as a snack
- Eat green leafy vegetables for the salad and avoid high fat/high caloric salad dressings
- Eat berries (strawberries, blueberries, raspberries, blackberries, etc.) fresh or frozen
- Eat an orange instead of drinking a glass of orange juice
- Avoid fried foods

Behavior #4: Read and Understand Nutrition Facts Labels

How many of you know how to read the nutrition label on the packaging of canned food, boxed food, or frozen meals? And if you do know how to read the label, do you understand what you're reading?

For example, do you realize there is a difference between a serving size and a portion?

You'll learn more about reading and understanding Nutrition Facts labels in a future chapter.

Behavior #5: Reduce Portion Sizes

Use a salad plate instead of a dinner plate. If you put the exact amount of food on a salad plate as on a dinner plate, the food on the dinner plate will look like you're getting less, and the food on the salad plate will look like you're getting more. It's an optical illusion. It's known as the Delboeuf Illusion.

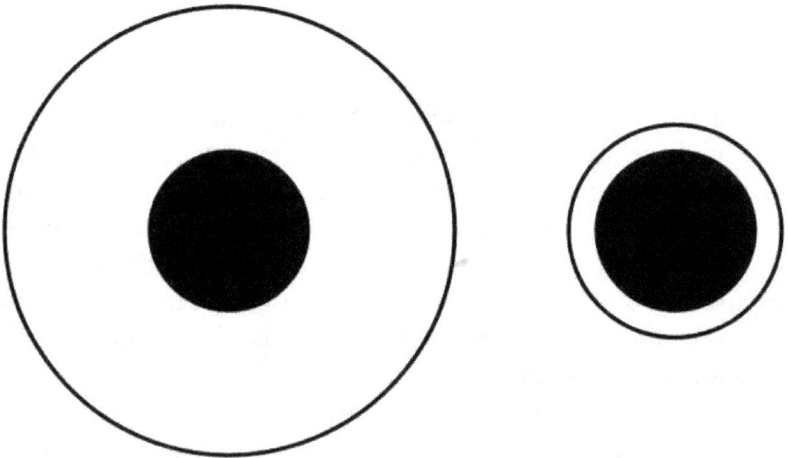

Franz Joseph Delboeuf, a Belgian mathematician and philosopher, first documented this phenomenon in 1865. Delboeuf started with two dots of equal size. He surrounded one dot with a large circle and the other dot with a small one. He noticed the second dot looked bigger.

Research suggests that choices, like how much to eat during a meal, are often made subconsciously. The problem arises because our brains are hard-wired to mislead us in lots of little ways, which can have a big impact on our diets.

Brian Wansink and Koert Van Ittersum, professors of marketing at Georgia Institute of Technology, performed a series of experiments and tests to measure the effect of the Delboeuf illusion on serving behavior and perceptions of serving size. Their work appeared in the *Journal of Consumer Research.* Wansink and Van Ittersum found that a dinner plate size significantly impacts food consumption. The professors asked Georgia Tech students to do various tasks of serving food. In one test, the students were to serve the same diameter (which represented the black dot in the center of the Delboeuf diagram) onto dinner plates of varying sizes, which represented the outer circles of Delboeuf's diagram.

What they found was the students served more food on the larger plates. They repeatedly under-served onto the smaller plates and over-served onto the larger ones. The students were unaware that they were doing this. The results demonstrated that the size of dinnerware you use to serve yourself on a day-to-day basis may significantly influence how much food you consume.

Van Ittersum said, "We are oftentimes our own worst enemy. And that's not because we want to overeat." Van Ittersum said that the illusion is embedded so deeply in our brains it is nearly impossible to overcome. Even telling test subjects about it ahead of time, as they did in another phase of the research, didn't eliminate the bias.

Other researchers also measured serving behavior in the real-world atmosphere of a buffet line. They found the same results. People underserved and overestimated on small dishes, while the reverse was true for large dishes. People using the smallest dishes undershot the target serving by as much as 12 percent. But people using the largest dishes took up to 13 percent more food than they intended.

According to Wansink and Van Ittersum, the average size of an American dinner plate has increased by almost 23 percent since 1900. In the '60s the average dinner plate was 9 inches in diameter and by the year 2000, it was 11 inches. Perhaps this is one of the reasons that the United States has a weight problem.

Restaurants are notorious for giving portions that are two or three times more than what we should be eating. So, what can you do when the server brings you your food that is too much to eat at one sitting? Simply cut it in half and ask for a to-go-box. Put one-half in the to-go-box. This will help you from overeating. Plus, you'll save money. It's like getting two meals for the price of one.

These are magic words you can use when eating at a restaurant. Inform the server, "I am on a restricted diet. I'd like to order... a plain grilled chicken breast with a side of avocado" or "a grilled salmon with a side of steamed broccoli" or "a grilled steak (6 ounces or smaller) with a side of plain green beans/mixed green salad (with dressing on the side)," etc. Every time I've done this, the server has been more than willing to accommodate my request.

Here's some food for thought, no pun intended. It's been scientifically proven that the size of your dinnerware affects your behavior for how much food you consume. If you increase your caloric intake by just 50 calories per day because you're eating more than you should, you will gain an additional five pounds within one year. This is how the weight creeps up on us. It's gradual over a long period of time. Imagine reversing that trend and eating less simply by using a smaller plate. You'd most likely reduce your caloric intake by 50 calories per day. Which means that over time you'd get rid of extra weight.

As you will recall, we demonstrated that if you shed just two pounds per month for 12 consecutive months, you'd weigh 24 pounds less within one year. The opposite holds true.

Behavior #6: Eat Slower

Do you eat your food fast?

Or, do you eat slow?

There's value to eating slowly. Learning to eat slower is one of the simplest yet most powerful things you can do to improve your overall health. We're all rushed, distracted, and too busy. Most people in the United States eat fast. Really fast. Rarely do people take the time to savor their food - or sometimes even to chew it properly. I know, I was like that. My nickname in college was turbo, short for turbocharger because I ate so fast.

Eating slower allows your body time to recognize that you're full. It takes about 20 minutes from the time you start to ingest your meal for the brain to signal you that you're satisfied. Most meals don't even last that long. As we learned in the previous lesson, our food is scientifically engineered such that our brain never gets the signal to stop eating.

Eating slowly helps you feel satisfied before overeating. Imagine the extra calories, sugars, carbs and fats you could eliminate simply by eating slower. Marc David, the author of *The Slow Down Diet,* suggests if you eat breakfast in five minutes, increase the time to 10. If you normally take 10 minutes, increase it to 15 or 20. Give yourself a minimum of 30-minutes (half-an-hour) for lunch and dinner.

The benefits of eating your food slower include better digestion, better hydration, easier weight loss or maintenance, and greater satisfaction with our meals. Meanwhile, eating quickly leads to poor digestion, increased weight gain, and lower satisfaction. The message is clear: Slow down your eating and enjoy improved health and well-being.

Shoveling down your food means that you can sneak in a lot of extra calories before your stomach realizes what is going on. At the University of Rhode Island, researchers examined how eating speed affected the early stages of digestive processing by observing 60 young adults eat a meal. What they found is:

- Slow eaters consumed 2 ounces of food per minute.
- Medium-speed eaters consumed 2.5 ounces of food per minute.
- Fast eaters consumed 3.1 ounces per minute. They also took larger bites and chewed less before swallowing.

In another University of Rhode Island study, researchers served lunch on two different occasions to 30 normal-weight women. When the researchers compared the difference in food consumption between the quickly eaten lunch and the slowly eaten lunch, here is what they found:

- When eating quickly, women consumed 646 calories in 9 minutes.
- When eating slowly, women consumed 579 calories in 29 minutes.

That is 67 *fewer* calories in 20 *more* minutes! For one meal.

If you extrapolate that to three meals per day, you can see how quickly those extra calories could add up. And here's another interesting twist: When the women ate their lunch quickly, they reported more hunger an hour later than those who ate their lunch slowly. So not only did eating quickly lead to greater food consumption, it satisfied the women *less*.

Conversely, of course, eating slower meant less food yet longer-lasting satisfaction. Who knew?

Here are a few suggestions to help you slow down your eating behavior:

- Put the fork or spoon down between each bite.
- Avoid eating while driving.
- Avoid eating while working or at your desk.
- Avoid eating while watching television.
- Focus on eating and enjoying your food.
- Avoid distractions while eating

As best you can, enroll your family, co-workers, and boss in creating more time and relaxation with meals. Find a "slow down" buddy to share meals and encourage each other to slow down while eating.

Eat only in a sitting position. Choose not to answer your cell phone, home phone, or texts while you're eating your food. When you slow down, savor a meal, pay attention to tastes and textures, and appreciate each mindful bite. This one small adjustment to your current eating routine can help you lose weight.

That reminds me of a story of when I ate fast. When I was in high school, my twin brother Larry, our friend Warren, and I sat down for lunch. My Mom had just served Warren and Larry their food. My brother asked, "Aren't you going to give David his food?"

To which my mother responded, "I did. He ate it already."

Although we all sat down together to eat, I had cleaned my plate before Warren and Larry had a chance to get their food. It wasn't like I ate my food, it was more like I inhaled it.

Can I share with you another example?

Great.

During my first year in college, about twice a week, a group of us played cards and ordered in pizza. Soon after we had a routine of playing, my roommate and friends suspected something wasn't quite right. One evening, after all the pizza had been eaten, Paul said, "I had only one slice, where's the rest?" Eric also said, "Hey, I only had one slice."

"Jim looked at them and said, "Don't look at me, I only had one."

Jay shook his head, looked at me and asked, "David how many slices did you eat?"

Sheepishly, I replied, "I guess I had the rest." It was about five slices of an extra-large pizza.

After that, they limited me to two slices.

During my sophomore year, while dining in the cafeteria, I had six plates of spaghetti within 10 minutes. The girl serving the food in the cafeteria asked me on the sixth serving, "Are you eating this or dumping it?"

"I'm eating it," I responded.

She just shook her head.

About 20 minutes later I ran three miles. Surprisingly, I kept the food down.

A fraternity brother pinned the nickname Turbo on me because, as he put it, I ate so fast, I acted like a turbocharged engine guzzling gas.

Despite my poor eating habits, I weighed 155 pounds. I got away with eating a lot of food quickly because I exercised a lot. Can you relate to this?

While in college, I went to a restaurant to celebrate a friend's birthday. I ordered the lobster tail. To my friends' amazement, I finished my meal last. They asked me if I was sick or felt ill. I said, "No, I wanted to enjoy it."

The point of this story is that I had the ability to eat leisurely, but I chose not to do so at all other times. If you make a conscious decision, you can eat slower. Yes, you can adapt and modify your eating behaviors. I'm a perfect example.

Behavior #7: Reduce and/or Avoid Alcoholic Beverages

Do you think drinking alcohol will cause you to gain weight? Or, are you of the opinion that consuming alcohol won't cause weight gain? Either answer is correct because it depends on the situation.

Drinking in moderation is usually considered OK from a health perspective, but it's important to really have a full grasp of just what "in moderation" means.

Are you aware that drinking in moderation refers to no more than one drink a day if you're a woman and no more than two a day for men? If you're drinking more than this, it could be considered problematic.

Alcohol can cause weight gain simply because it has calories. Not only does the alcohol have calories, but additives and mixers that are included with many alcoholic beverages can be packed with calories as well as sugar. The calories that come from alcohol are considered empty, meaning they have no nutritional value. If you have too much alcohol, it can also turn into fat in your liver, which then turns into fat in your blood and is likely to be stored as fat in your body.

The Foundation for Alcohol Research and Education conducted a study on alcohol and obesity that found:

- It is unclear whether alcohol consumption is a risk factor for weight gain because studies performed to date have found positive, negative, or no association.
- Where there is a positive association between alcohol and body weight it is more likely to be found in men than in women.

- The present data provide inadequate scientific evidence to assess whether beer intake is associated with general or abdominal obesity.
- When considering beer, where there is a positive association, it is more likely to be for abdominal obesity (abdominal fat around the stomach) than for general obesity for men and women.

So yes, it's possible to gain weight from alcohol, but it's not inevitable.

Whether or not you personally gain weight from drinking alcohol depends on many factors. These include:

- Your behaviors when you drink
- What you drink
- How often you drink
- How much you drink
- What you eat when you drink
- Factors that relate to your unique body and lifestyle
- Your overall diet
- Your genetics
- Your gender
- Your level of physical activity
- Your age

Some suggestions to accomplish behavior change include, but not limited to:

1. Avoid drinking beer or wine.
2. If unable to avoid consuming alcohol, drink one beer or half a glass of wine.
3. Avoid all hard liquor.

Behavior #8: Watch Your Thoughts, Watch Your Words – They Have Impact

Watch your thoughts. Watch your words. They have an impact. You are not making a sacrifice by avoiding certain foods. You're making a choice. You are not depriving yourself of sweets, ice cream, cookies, cakes, etc. You're making a choice. Remember, we all make choices. Think positively. Think in terms of releasing weight, rather than losing weight. Think in terms of reducing weight, not losing weight. When you lose something, you tend to want to find it. You are not foregoing that piece of pumpkin pie or pecan pie. You are making a choice not to indulge.

Behavior #9: Stop Eating at Least Three Hours Before You Go to Sleep

Do you eat after 7:00 p.m.?

Do you have late night snacks or eat just prior to going to bed?

Can we agree there is no universal time that everyone should stop eating? After all, we all get up at different times, go to sleep at different times, and have other reasons, such as business meetings, social events, or dating to eat at different times.

But. if you are reducing weight, do <u>NOT</u> eat or drink anything, except pure water, at least three hours between the time you eat dinner or a healthy dessert and the time you go to sleep.

Why is this important?

According to some experts, restricting your food intake from 6:00 a.m. to 7:00 p.m. can reduce the overall calorie intake drastically. Further, a longer duration of overnight fast helps with increasing fat loss because the body has time to reach a state of ketosis - a natural state for the body, when it is almost completely fueled by fat.

What this means for you is your body is using stored fat for energy. Researchers from the Perelman School of Medicine at the University of Pennsylvania found that eating late at night has some negative effects on your overall health. They found evidence that eating late at night raises glucose and insulin levels, both of which are causes of Type 2 diabetes. This new study has suggested that snacking late at night could increase your risk of diabetes and heart disease.

The evidence suggested that poor timing of meals can also raise cholesterol levels which can increase the risk of heart disease or suffering a heart attack. Researchers from Dokuz Eylül University in Turkey found that eating after 7:00 p.m. could increase the risk for you to have a heart attack. They assessed more than 700 adults with high blood pressure in order to find out whether different eating times made a difference in their health.

The information gleaned from the study also indicated that eating dinner late at night had the most significant impact on overnight blood pressure while eating within two hours of going to sleep did more damage than indulging in a high salt content diet. According to the research, 24.2 percent of those who ate dinner within two hours of going to bed suffered from high blood pressure which did not drop sufficiently overnight, compared with 14.2 percent of those who ate their evening meal at least three hours earlier.

Further, another study done by researchers at the University of California found that eating at irregular hours - such as late at night - had the potential to impact cognitive functions. Dr. Jamie Koufman is a New York Times bestselling author of several books about acid reflux and has been listed as one of "America's Top Doctors" every year since 1994. He says going to sleep shortly after eating late at night (especially heavy foods) is a key contributor to acid reflux.

Dr. Kaufman explains that it takes your stomach a few hours to empty after a meal. So, when you go to sleep shortly after eating, it allows for the acid to spill out of your still full stomach and leak into your esophagus, leading to acid reflux. Speaking to The New York Times in 2014, Kaufman said, "The drugs we are using to treat reflux don't always work, and even when they do, they can have dangerous side effects. Dr. Kaufman also stated, "My patient's reflux was a lifestyle problem. I told him he had to eat dinner before 7:00 p.m., and not eat at all after work. Within six weeks, his reflux was gone."

Do you get up in the middle of the night to raid the refrigerator?

Another consequence of eating late at night is it can have you feeling hungrier than usual when you wake up the next morning. The reason being that the insulin your pancreas releases after a meal, which in turn produces more glucose, which triggers a hormone called ghrelin. Ghrelin is responsible for triggering hunger. Ghrelin normally resets itself between around 8:00 p.m. to 8:00 a.m.

Some of the challenges you might face if attempting to not eat after 7:00 p.m. or at least three hours before going to sleep are:

- Going out to dinner with friends. If you go out with other couples, do you frequently often eat after 8:00 p.m. or later?
- Do you have business meetings, workshops, or seminars that make it difficult, if not impossible to eat earlier?

There's not much you can do in these situations. But it's the other times when we eat at home that we can improve our habit and behaviors when we eat our meals. One component to successful weight reduction is to eliminate eating or drinking anything three hours before you turn in for the night. Most weight-loss experts agree you should refrain from eating at least three hours before bedtime.

Maybe being aware of this can help you improve so that you avoid eating or snacking at least three hours before going to sleep.

Behavior #10: Get Adequate Sleep

Do you feel you get adequate sleep each night?

Or do you know you're not getting enough sleep?

Researchers have found that getting adequate sleep each night is a basic principle for maintaining good health and lowering your risk of gaining weight.

Why?

Because not getting the proper amount of sleep elevates your cortisol levels. Cortisol causes your body to go into fat storage mode. Elevated cortisol levels cause junk food cravings. And, not having enough sleep makes you tired, which increases your cravings for junk food. You'll know if you're tired all the time because you'll also be hungry all the time.

Getting adequate sleep is crucial for reducing weight. Getting enough sleep is required for turning off fat retention programs, reducing stress, reducing cortisol levels, and maintaining proper hormonal balance.

It is better, for weight-loss purposes, to take a nap in the afternoon instead of exercising or working out. That is, you will lose more weight by taking a nap in mid-afternoon that you will if you work out. I know it sounds contradictory to what we've been taught, but if you are sleep deprived, it's better to take a nap. Nothing is more important that getting the proper amount of sleep when you're tired when you're attempting to reduce weight.

Suggestions to accomplish behavior change for sleeping better at night:
1. Turn your computer screens off an hour before bedtime.
2. Turn your television off an hour before bedtime.
3. Turn your WiFi on your phone off at bedtime.
4. Put your phone on airplane mode.
5. Reduce as much light as possible. Make the room as dark as possible.
6. Keep the room cool. Studies show that when a room is cool you sleep better.

Let's Recap
The 10 eating behaviors to change and improve are:
1. Drink more water
2. Avoid processed foods
3. Eat whole or holistic foods
4. Read and understand nutrition labels
5. Reduce portion sizes
6. Eat slower
7. Reduce or avoid alcoholic beverages
8. Watch your thoughts, watch your words -they have impact
9. Stop eating at least three hours before going to sleep
10. Get adequate sleep

Now you know what to do, and how to improve your eating behavior. The only question is, will you?

"NO" is a Choice
There is a secret to achieving a healthy weight and lifestyle. The answer is one word. That one word is "No."

The only way to win against your willpower, self-control, and discipline for reducing weight is not to play. When you choose not to play, you win by default. This is what I mean. If you're attempting to reduce weight, willpower, self-control, and discipline will fail you 100 percent of the time.

In this day and age, to reduce weight in a healthy and sustainable manner you need insane focus to counteract the onslaught of the crazy distractions and temptations working against you. These factions and factors include TV ads for food and restaurants, other people in your life, social occasions, special events, and holidays. You must create focused, guarded boundaries.

Would you like to eliminate refined sugars, bread, muffins, cake, and 90 percent of the Standard American Diet (S.A.D.) and never waffle or waiver? Whatever situation you find yourself in won't matter. Be it birthday parties, holidays, special occasions, company functions, social gatherings, there is an absolute rule. That rule is under no circumstances will you answer anything but "No" or "No thank you," when offered something you know you shouldn't eat.

Just don't give in. Don't do it. Treat it like a pregnant woman does alcohol. For a pregnant woman, when offered alcohol, the answer should always be "No." Or take someone who has an allergy to food such as nuts. When asked if they will make an exception to eating a few nuts or products made with nuts, the answer for them is always, "No." No matter what. Beware of making exceptions because they tend to become the rule.

Make the choice once. If you make the choice once not to indulge in eating refined sugar, processed foods, cakes, pie, doughnuts, ice cream, sweets, bread, snacks such as chips, crackers, or pretzels, then you never need to make it again. You'll reduce a thousand choices into one. The choice not to eat chips, pretzels, cookies, sweets, processed foods, etc. is yours.

You'll avoid all those situational, conditional, well/but circumstances that collapse on you every time to challenge (and win) over your willpower, discipline, and self-control. You've already made the decision and the answer will be, "No, I choose not to indulge or partake."

You eliminate the need to make a choice because the choice has already been made. It's a hard and fast rule of absolutely, "No." No if's, but's, or exceptions, and no need to re-think the decision every time in every circumstance and situation.

Do you have the character to draw the proverbial "hard line" in the sand? We shall see. Your waistline will be the determination if you succeed.

Cash Out at the End of the Day

Cash out at the end of the day based on what you inputted (what you said you were going to do) versus what you put out (what you did). Cash out every day by reviewing what you said you were going to do and at the end of the day what you did. Did you do it? Or did you not?

For example, did you say you would refrain from drinking soda/diet soda and drink pure water? If so, did you drink a minimum of 64 ounces of pure water throughout the day? Keep track of this daily.

At the end of the week are you on track or are you off track? This is your gyroscope. No matter what weight you start at, you can end up exactly the weight you intend to be if you keep yourself on track all along the way. "What doesn't get measured, doesn't get done." – Darren Hardy

In the next chapter, you'll learn how changing and improving your mindset can help you to reduce weight.

Chapter 5

Mindset to Achieve and Maintain a Healthy Weight

The ultimate measure of a man [person] is not where he [she] stands in the moment of comfort and convenience, but where he [she] stands at times of challenge.

Dr. Martin Luther King

D o you have a personal Code of Honor?
I'm guessing you probably don't.

Do you work for a company that has a Code of Honor?

A Code of Honor is a set of rules which you and others agree to abide by. It is your principles or a way of life. Without rules, people make up their own.

In this chapter, you will learn why it's important to have a personal Code of Honor for your weight-reduction journey, the importance of thinking in positive terms for weight-reduction, the mental, emotional, and psychological aspects of losing weight in a healthy and sustainable manner and using gratitude to reduce weight.

Thousands of books have been written about diet, weight loss, nutrition, fitness, and exercise. There are numerous weight-loss programs advertised on television, radio, and the internet. At the grocery store checkout, you'll see hundreds of new ideas to lose weight touted on the front covers of magazines. Yet, more than 71 percent of the U.S. adult population is overweight.

How many of you have heard of or have been on the...

- Paleo diet?
- Keto diet?
- Mediterranean diet?
- South Beach diet?

- Jenny Craig?
- Weight Watchers?
- Nutrisystem?
- Medifast?
- HCG, like myself?
- The Atkins Diet?
- The Vegan Diet?
- The Zone Diet?
- The Ultra Low-Fat Diet?

Wow, that's a lot of types of diets. The one thing most have in common – they ignore a powerful tool: A Code of Honor.

In his book, **Team Code of Honor – The Secrets of Champions in Business and Life,** author Blair Singer states,

> *Those who are successful have a very clear Code of Honor that is easy to understand and is not negotiable or subject to interpretations. It's a strong set of rules that everyone around them agrees to and part of what makes everyone around them successful as well.*

To succeed in any weight-reduction program, you'll need a Code of Honor, to have rules, to be held accountable and to have support from others. Make your family, friends, co-workers, colleagues and even your doctor a part of your team to support your weight-reduction journey.

Although shedding your extra pounds is something you must do yourself, it doesn't mean you have to do it alone. It helps to have a support team to keep you accountable. No one said getting rid of weight is easy. It's not. If someone tells you it is easy, run, because they are lying.

Do you **wish** you could drop a few pounds?

Do you **want** to shed a few pounds?

There's a difference between wishing or wanting something to happen and doing something to make it happen. Execution separates the wishers in life from the successful people who act. People who care enough about their lives and future to do something instead of hoping it will happen. They act.

Have you thought about shedding a few extra pounds? Maybe talked about doing something about it? But, what efforts have you made to get rid of those unwanted extra pounds?

"I'd do anything to lose 15 pounds, except eat healthy, drink more water, give up wine or beer, and start exercising." Does this sound like you? I've met hundreds of people who say they ***want*** to lose weight, but they're just not willing to do anything about it or make changes to their lifestyle. It's time to get out of your comfort zone.

Your Code of Honor reflects you and your standards. Your waistline will determine if you're abiding by your code. Share your code with others. If they are willing to abide by your code, and they agree with it, great.

If they disagree with it or aren't on board and willing to help you stick to your code, they may be the wrong fit for you. You might consider re-evaluating your relationship with the people who don't or won't support you.

People without a support team or someone to hold them accountable tend to give up on weight-reduction programs. It is difficult to have a spouse or significant other eating pizza, pasta, or desserts while you're trying to improve your eating habits. Most people, with few exceptions, need to have someone to check in with to keep them accountable and stay on track.

If you can't find someone to join you on your weight-reduction journey, join or create a weight-reduction meetup group. Having a community that encourages you or one-on-one accountability partner or coach is invaluable.

Your weight reduction Code of Honor is the set of rules *you* agreed to. Every person has their own rules, their own Code of Honor. Therefore, it's imperative that you make sure everyone understands *your* Code of Honor and that you want to play by the rules defined in it and that they must too.

Marines have a strict Code of Honor. They need to be rigid because when bullets start buzzing by a person's head, emotion tends to elevate and intelligence decreases. The code is drilled into Marines over and over to keep them together under pressure. It's a matter of life and death. Otherwise, individuals won't do the right thing to protect the team, the mission and each other.

I'm not saying being in battle is the same or even close to being anything like being in battle when it comes to reducing weight, but for some of you, it can be a matter of life and death. For others, it could make a difference between enjoying life or living in misery.

Honor your code. Respect the code of others.

Here are examples of what you might want to include in your Code of Honor. You can choose which rules you want to adopt as yours or you can create your own.

1. Mission. The mission I have chosen is to reduce weight in a healthy manner and to keep it off!
2. Be accountable.
3. Adjust my relationship with food to ensure it is viewed as fuel for my body and not as comfort from my emotions.
4. Record everything, I ingest in a daily journal.
5. Commit to learning about nutrition and better eating habits.
6. Commit to a lifestyle change.
7. Never impose my standards on anyone else.
8. Never blame others for my failures. I will take 100 percent responsibility for my own success. No justifications. I'll either have excuses or results.
9. Be willing to get called out if I violate the code. My team (support group and/or coach) must be willing to enforce the code.
10. Never judge or pre-judge others.
11. Motivate, encourage, and empower others to lose weight, but only if they have a desire to do so.
12. Do not seek sympathy or acknowledgment. I want to reduce weight and keep it off for me. Not anyone else. No one can do it for me. I must be willing to do it myself.
13. Note: It's great if you, the reader, have a purpose or reason, some call it "the why," for wanting to lose weight. But the bottom line is that it's your choice.
14. Don't compare yourself to others. We're all unique; we all have our special gifts.

15. Do not compete with others. Complete others.

16. Be a role model for others.

If you want, add more of what's important to you. Take some time to reflect on what's important to you to reduce your weight and keep it off. Share your thoughts and ideas with others before finalizing it. Once you do finalize your Code of Honor, it should not be modified, unless under extreme circumstances.

Many overweight individuals tend to blame others for their problem with weight. You must be accountable for your own weight issues. Therefore, it's important to have a Code of Honor to keep you accountable. Jillian Michaels, trainer on the NBC TV hit show, *Biggest Loser*, says, "Don't blame anyone or anything for your situation or problems. When you do that, you are saying that you are powerless over your own life – which is utter crap. An empowering step to reclaiming your life is taking responsibility." Be accountable and responsible for your own issues. You are not powerless. Take charge of your life.

Think in positive terms for weight reduction; the mental, emotional, and psychological aspects of losing weight in a healthy and sustainable manner are important. It's not always what you're eating but what you're saying or thinking to yourself. If you've had thoughts or have said, "I've tried everything. No matter what I do, I can't lose weight." that is being negative.

Can you relate to this?

Our minds are the most important part of the body for weight reduction, but it is the one area most weight-loss programs ignore or neglect. Your greatest enemy for reducing weight and shedding those unwanted pounds lives between your ears. Your success in reducing weight begins when you change your mindset. Sandra Yancey, CEO, and Founder of the eWomenNetwork, said, "If you want to change what's visible, you need to change what's invisible – your mindset." Sam Milman said, "Thinking about doing something is the same as doing nothing." The same applies to reducing weight. Just thinking about losing weight and not acting is the same as doing nothing to make it happen. Buddha said, "All that we are is the result of what we have thought. The mind is everything. What we think we become."

Your desire to get rid of weight is based on a combination of your thoughts, your feelings, and how those affect your eating habits and actions. This is your mindset. Your feelings lead to your emotions. Your emotions control your thoughts. Your thoughts control your actions. Your actions lead to your temperament. Your temperament determines your behavior, which predicts your results.

Mastering your behavior is paramount to your weight-reduction success. And it all begins with your mindset. Have you wondered why it's so difficult to improve our eating habits? We all know what to do, we just don't do it. The source of being overweight is poor eating habits based on poor choices. But why do you make poor choices? Perhaps, it's not so much of the poor choices we make, but our flawed relationship with food. It's from the way we think about food.

Many people turn to food for comfort if they're having a bad day, are hurt or upset. Do you? In movies or TV shows, when someone is upset or hurt, the first thing they show is that person eating a pint of ice cream or stuffing cookies or cake into their mouths.

Many people enjoy the food at social gatherings, holidays, and special occasions such as birthdays and anniversaries. Rarely, if ever, do people think about food as fuel and nutrition for your bodies. Perhaps we just don't care.

The obvious answer to improving our eating habits is to change our thinking about why we eat, what we're eating, when we eat, and how we're eating. Getting rid of the stinking thinking is easy to say, but not so easy to do. Unfortunately, too many of us have negative thoughts that are non-supportive, not just for weight loss, but most everything else in life.

Humans have between 12,000 to 60,000 thoughts per day. According to some research, as many as 98 percent of them are exactly ones you had the day before. Talk about creatures of habit! Even more significant, 80 percent of our thoughts are negative. Imagine that – 80 percent of our thoughts are negative and non-supportive.

Take a moment to contemplate what your life would be like if your thought process was reversed and 80 percent of your thoughts were positive and supportive.

Psychoneuroimmunology is the medical term for the mind/body connection. You've experienced it. We all have. If you've been doing mental work all day, you're likely to feel tired physically, too. Do you come home from work feeling exhausted even though you did not do any physical activity? Contrarily, if you're tired from physical activity, such as manual labor, do you find it difficult to think clearly and focus? That's because there is a direct correlation between how your body feels as it relates to your mind and vice versa.

Negative thoughts are especially draining. Thoughts containing words like "never," "should," and "can't," complaints, whining, or thoughts that diminish your own or another's sense of self-worth deplete the body by producing corresponding chemicals that weaken the physiology.

The good news is, if you can recognize a negative or limiting thought, you can consciously choose to change it. Instead of saying, "I can't lose weight," say, "I have the power to control my weight. I have a strong urge to eat healthy foods and forgo processed foods." The chemicals produced by your body as a response to this kind of thought are more likely to support you in fulfilling your goal.

The only way to override the negative and non-supportive thinking is with positive and supportive thoughts. What you focus on expands. Oprah Winfrey is credited with saying, "What you focus on expands, and when you focus on the goodness in your life, you create more of it."

Negative thinking will never make your life positive because a negative mind will never give you a positive life.

Rumi, the 13th-century poet, mystic, and scholar said, "What you seek is seeking you." Are you seeking to modify and improve your eating behaviors?

You get what you focus on. So, focus on what you want, not what you don't want. That is the Law of Attraction. With respect to weight reduction, too many are more focused on being overweight and needing to reduce weight than on the solutions to their overweight issues.

If you're focusing on the fact that you're overweight or fat, then that is what life will keep serving you. In the weight-loss game, those who focus on the problem rather than the solution, get more problems.

Eventually, you may have an under-active thyroid, maybe you become insulin resistant or some other hormonal issue. These are excuses and reasons people use to justify their weight-loss failures. People who lose weight and get into their ideal shape are focused on the solution. They believe in attaining their goal. They want it and their actions are reflective of their belief. They look for ways to improve rather than reasons why they can't.

The problem for many, especially those who have never really tasted success or know anything else but being overweight is that their belief in themselves reaching their goal is low to non-existent. Their self-esteem sucks. They have terrible, negative, non-supportive self-talk.

Stop looking outside of you. Everything you need to be successful exists within the space between your ears. You most likely don't need a different gym membership, you don't need a new supplement, and you don't need to follow a new diet. You need to back yourself and BELIEVE! Use affirmations and visualizations as a tool to program your mind to believe and then take consistent and persistent action based on those thoughts.

Stop lying in B.E.D!

B.E.D is Blame – Excuses – Denial. Take responsibility for your thoughts, acknowledge when your self-talk is negative and then aim to steer your thoughts in a more positive direction. Focus on what you can control and then go take some action based on those thoughts. Realize that your state of consciousness creates your reality and your reality is yours to make whatever you so choose.

It's imperative that you create the thoughts you want about food and put them on autopilot, so they become second nature and natural. Do it to a point so that your thoughts are no longer negative but are positive. Your positive thinking becomes as normal as brushing your teeth.

If you don't learn to manage your way of thinking about food, you are doomed to a life-based on failure and struggle with weight issues. Your old concepts about food will keep you stuck. Consciousness is observing your thoughts and actions so that you can live from true decision-making in the present moment rather than being run by programming from the past.

Let me give you an example. You're at your grandmother's home and just finished a fine meal. Grandma brings out one of her world-famous pecan pies. She knows you want to lose weight. So, she gives you a choice. You can have a piece of the delicious mouth-watering pie or a glass of water.

If you choose the pie, you get immediate joy and satisfaction, an awesome sense of pleasure because the pecan pie is amazing. If you choose the glass of water, you get nothing. And, if the others who joined you for dinner at Grandma's choose the pie, you might feel some anger or resentment. This is the challenge you face. Not just at Grandma's, but every day, all day.

If you make a poor choice by selecting the pie, you're immediately rewarded. You have instantaneous gratification. If you make a good choice, a healthy choice, you get nothing. And that's what you'll be fighting day-in and day-out. You're fighting against your own mind.

You'll be bombarded with a gauntlet of images and smells designed to increase your cravings and temptations all day long. Your ability to stay focused and disciplined will be challenged by television ads for restaurants, foods, pizza, fried chicken, tempting desserts, snacks, candy, and other things. You'll pass by numerous signs and billboards promoting fast food establishments. Not to mention the occasional office party or get together with friends.

Here's the paradox. What gives you the short term, instant gratification and pleasure, such as the pecan pie or other foods and beverages, most likely causes you pain and suffering in the long run. You'll be at a higher risk of developing chronic illnesses and diseases such as Type 2 diabetes, different forms of cancer, possible liver disease, and an increased risk for a heart attack or stroke. The other side is that what causes resentment and possible pain, such as choosing to not eat the pie or other desserts, in the short term will reward you in the long term with a higher probability for maintaining a healthy weight and better health.

According to Darren Hardy, in life, you'll "suffer" two types of pain. You get to choose your pain. You can choose the pain of regret or the pain of being disciplined. Hardy said, "The pain of discipline weighs ounces. The pain of regret weighs tons." It's not easy to make a healthier choice. But, it's a lot less painful if the choice of regret is that you do suffer a heart attack, stroke, or contract a chronic illness or disease. The fundamentals of achieving and maintaining a healthy weight are easy: eat holistic (whole) foods, mostly plants, not too much, avoid processed foods, drink lots of pure water, and get proper rest. These, unfortunately, are the most often ignored.

It's an internal fight about being consistent. T. Harv Eker said, "How you do anything is how you do everything." Similarly, Dave Ramsey said, "If you live like no one else, later you can live like no one else." Of course, Dave Ramsey was talking about financial advice. But the same can be applied to achieving and maintaining a healthy weight. If you eat like no one else, i.e., avoid fast foods and processed foods, and eat primarily whole/holistic foods, you'll most likely enjoy good health where others will suffer from chronic illnesses.

It bears repeating. reducing weight is a state of mind. Either you control your thoughts, or they control you. Either way, it's your choice. Training and managing your mindset are the most important skills you can learn in terms of both happiness and success. It's doable and you can do it.

Weight-loss programs tend to be a temporary solution because they're incomplete. They don't help people change their thought process or their relationship with food. There is a lot of empirical evidence and data that proves the majority of those who lose weight fail to keep it off. They gain the weight back.

Teaching you how to make improvements and changes to your thinking to improve your eating behavior and habits is extremely important and critical for successfully achieving and maintaining a healthy weight.

What will motivate you to reduce your weight? Or, if this doesn't apply to you, what will motivate someone you know or love who should shed a few pounds, or more, but won't? Anthony Trucks is credited with saying, "The fact that you aren't the weight you want to be should be enough motivation." Unfortunately, for most of you, it's not.

Each of us has our own word, image, sound or something that will trigger us to want to slim down. For my friends Henry and Robert, the word "diabetes" scared them so much they finally made a commitment to shed their extra pounds. For other friends, it was being worried about their emerging heart problems. For me, it was my doctor telling me, "Lose weight, or you will die."

The number one reason people decide to lose weight is for health reasons. The second most cited reason for reducing weight is to improve appearances. For others, it might be wanting to look good for a special event, such as a wedding, class reunion, or family photo. Or, it may be not wanting to take your shirt off in a pick-up basketball game.

Your motivation to reduce weight must be impactful enough for you not to just want it, but to act, and then follow through. Are you doing it for your children or grandkids? It's up to you to determine what will be that one thing to compel you to get rid of your extra weight, act, and then follow through. You'll need to want to lose weight so much so that you'll commit to it. You need a deep, intense, white-hot burning desire to conquer being overweight. Jim Rohn once said, "The bigger the why, the easier the how." If you have a compelling reason or good enough purpose for losing weight and keeping it off, how you'll get it done will come.

If you don't have a compelling reason to lose weight and change your lifestyle, consider this: diseases and medical ailments associated with being overweight include, but aren't limited to, Type 2 diabetes, heart disease, stroke, liver failure, high blood pressure, sleep apnea, osteoarthritis, certain cancers, and many more. Why would you want to wait until you contract a medical condition that could be avoided simply by improving your lifestyle? Keep in mind the old cliché, "An ounce of prevention is worth a pound of cure."

Remember, 70 percent of people hospitalized are there because of food-related issues that are preventable. More people are dying from complications of being overweight than from smoking. Seven out of every ten adults in the U.S. are overweight, of which four of them are clinically obese. Look around and notice how many of your friends, relatives, co-workers, colleagues, and acquaintances are overweight or obese.

Your mindset matters. Without changing your mindset about weight reduction and a willingness to change your eating habits, any attempt to lose weight and keep it off will be futile. Losing weight is hard. Staying fit and trim is hard, and it never stops. It's like running a marathon without a finish line. Staying fat and overweight is easy.

John F. Kennedy, during his speech at Rice University on September 12, 1962, challenged the American people by saying:

> "We choose to go to the moon. We choose to go to the moon in this decade and do other things, not because they are easy, but because they are hard; because that goal will serve to organize and measure the best of our energies and skills; because that challenge is one that we're willing to accept..."

You must choose to reduce your weight. You must choose to change your eating habits and lifestyle. Because if you do choose to reduce weight in a healthy and sustainable manner, it will, as Kennedy said, *"Organize and measure the best of [y]our energies and skills."*

Yesterday You Said Tomorrow

Are you a procrastinator?

Have you put off reducing weight because it wasn't the perfect time, or you struggled with it? Each day, countless numbers of people say they will start their diet tomorrow. Unfortunately, for most of them, tomorrow never comes. Many people will tell themselves, "I'll start Monday." Of course, when Monday rolls around, there's always an excuse for not starting.

Have you used the excuse, "I'll start after the holidays?" Or, maybe, "I'll start after our vacation." Perhaps, you told yourself, "I'll start after we meet our friends for dinner on Wednesday?"

The reality is there is no perfect time to start to improve and change your eating habits and lifestyle. The best advice I can offer you is, just start a weight-loss program and never stop. As Zig Ziglar so eloquently put it, "You don't have to be great to start, but you have to start to be great."

Nike had a message that really resonated with me: "Yesterday you said tomorrow." We all know that if we put off until tomorrow what we can do today, we are just kidding ourselves. Waiting to do something until tomorrow is another fallacy. More excuses, more justification to delay, until it may be too late. Please don't delay implementing a process to improve and modify your eating behaviors. Act now! You'll either keep making excuses, have reasons, or you'll have results.

If you wait until you feel like losing weight, you'll likely never accomplish it. Mark Twain stated it best when he said, "Don't wait. The time will never be just right." If you do start a regimen to improve your eating behavior and habits, be certain you are resolved and committed to following through. Half-hearted efforts never produce positive results. Art Williams wasn't talking about reducing weight when he said, "I'm not telling you it's going to be easy. I'm telling you it's going to be worth it." The same can be said about improving your eating behaviors and habits to lose weight. I can tell you it won't be easy, but it will be worth it.

What we focus on we create. Focus on what you want to create rather than what you want to avoid. Think positively. Watch your thoughts. Watch your words. They have an impact. You are not making a sacrifice by avoiding certain foods. You're making a choice. You are not depriving yourself of anything, i.e., sweets, ice cream, cookies, cakes, etc. You're making a choice. Remember, we all make choices. Think positively. Think in terms of releasing weight, rather than losing weight. Think in terms of reducing weight, not losing weight. As I said earlier, when you lose something, you tend to want to find it. You are not foregoing that piece of pumpkin pie or pecan pie. You are making a choice not to indulge.

I'm not telling you that you can never enjoy a piece of cake or pie or a scoop of ice cream. That is not realistic. If you do decide to indulge and enjoy some ice cream, cake or pie, only have a small amount. Have a spoonful of ice cream instead of a scoop, or two. Have a sliver of cake or pie. You don't have to eat an entire piece. This can satisfy your craving and not set you back on your weight-loss journey. No one is perfect. If you do overindulge, don't beat yourself up over it. Just keep moving forward.

By the same token, don't keep making excuses for making exceptions. Exceptions tend to become the rule. I'm talking about those little voices in your head telling you, "It's okay to eat that candy bar or cookie," or "You've earned that piece of pie or dessert." No! it's not OK to have that candy bar or eat that cookie. No! it's not OK to "treat" yourself if you're still attempting to lose weight.

Do you want to reduce weight and improve your eating habits or not? If so, what are you willing to improve and change to make it happen? We can all agree nothing about your weight will change if you're not willing to do something different.

It may sound like you're getting conflicting information. You are right. The point you need to understand is, it's not OK to overindulge eating things you know aren't going to help you lose weight. Those chips you're thinking of having, don't. But, every so often, if you do have some chips, it's not the end of the world. Just don't make it a new old habit.

Have you tried to lose weight before only to have someone tell you, "Have just one, it won't kill you?" Or, "One cookie won't hurt you." No, it won't hurt you. No, it won't kill you. But it will prevent you from accomplishing your goal of getting rid of your extra weight. Be polite, but respectfully decline. The word "no" is a complete sentence. Just say, "No, thank you." You do not need to give an explanation. Sometimes I'll tell someone, "It will look better on you than me."

There are many more variations of situations to make an exception so be wary. There will be those people who will tell you, "You can't lose weight, so just go ahead and eat." Or, "You won't be able to do it. So, why bother?" Maybe it's your own little voices telling you these negative thoughts? Or you've heard the statistic that 90 percent of those who start a diet fail? And of those that do succeed in dropping the pounds, 85 percent gain it all back. So, why bother?

Have you had those thoughts?

Don't believe them because they are the ones who can't. You can do it. Joel Weldon has an expression, "Success comes in cans, not in cannots." You are not dieting. You are improving and changing your eating habits. You are the 10 to 15 percent who can and will succeed in achieving a healthy weight and maintaining it. You are the exception because you are not participating in the new normal.

Sticking with your commitment is tough during holidays or going to restaurants for meals. At restaurants, these words will help you tremendously: "I'm on a restrictive diet... I'd like to order... (add in what you enjoy, whether it be grilled chicken, fish, or a steak) and a side of steamed vegetables." You'd be surprised how many servers want you to succeed.

Friends and family members might react differently. While they want you to succeed with your weight-loss efforts, they might feel slighted or offended. After all, they did go through the expense and trouble to prepare a holiday meal for you. Be resolved but be polite. The following words can help you. Consider saying them when you accept the invitation, not when you sit down at the table!

- I am watching my weight. Please do not be offended if I refuse the food you offer or are serving.
- Please do not ask me to make an exception. Generally, I have found that exceptions become the rule. This is one reason I am on a weight-reduction program. Surely, you will sympathize with my efforts.
- I hope you'll understand why I must refuse whatever you have so graciously prepared. Thank you so much for your support and cooperation, it means a lot to me.

Staying committed is the key to permanent weight reduction. That's why it's important to improve and modify your eating behaviors so they become new habits.

Cruises will test your resolve. So, will all-inclusive resorts. Can I give you a little example of this? When my wife and I were at an all-inclusive resort in the Caribbean, the buffet became a challenge. To avoid overeating, I choose to use a salad plate instead of a dinner size plate. I only took what I wanted to eat, not what I wanted to try. When I finished my first serving, I was done. I did not go back for a second, or third helping. I also declined alcoholic beverages and opted for black coffee or water with lemon and no ice instead. I made it a game to not overeat. I watched other people go back for second, third, and fourth helpings. It was fascinating to sit and watch others stuffing food into their mouths. Just because it's all you can eat doesn't mean you have to eat it all.

The most difficult person to negotiate with is ourselves. We have discussions with the little voices in our head, especially when it comes to reducing weight.

Jerzy Gregorek said, "Hard choices, easy life. Easy choices, hard life." Take a minute to soak that in because this is so true. Hard choices include forcing yourself to act. "Hard choices, easy life" applies to eating healthy now to be healthy later. You're not making a sacrifice by not eating the bread, by not eating the piece of cake or scoop of ice cream. You're not depriving yourself or foregoing anything. It's a choice. You're choosing to not eat whatever it is that's not healthy or helping you to reduce your weight. Hard choices are learning how to do something rather than just waiting for someone else to do it for you. It's being responsible for yourself. It's being accountable – to yourself.

Anyone and everyone can succeed in reducing weight. It comes down to your mind and the little voices we all have. We are all mentally weak when it comes to shedding weight. Our mind is what sabotages us the most. The epic battle of getting rid of your unwanted weight will be won defeating your own mind. Your body can do much more than your mind wants to allow. The toughest person to negotiate with is yourself. And your potential is much greater than your mind wants you to stretch and go for it. If you are not at the weight you want to be, I'm telling you it's your mind's fault. The reason your mind sabotages your efforts to reduce weight and keep it off is one reason – survival. Survival at all costs. When your survival is threatened, your mind can tap into your raw, awesome potential that you had inside you all along. Outside of survival mode, the mind is weak.

To be more mentally tough when it comes to eating and food choices, scare your brain straight with a threat. Fear is your friend when it comes to stimulating your mind.

Make sure your worst enemy isn't the one residing between your own two ears. It's how you manage that conversation that will determine your success or failure.

Do you use declarations each day?

Do you use affirmations each day? Declarations are different from affirmations.

A declaration is stating the objective of doing something. Whereas, an affirmation states that a goal is already happening. This might not be true for your weight-reduction, in which case, your mind will immediately dismiss this statement.

An affirmation is basically just self-talk. It's a statement about ourselves or our situation that's phrased in the present tense as if the self-focused declaration is already true. We continually use affirmations subconsciously with words and thoughts and this flow of affirmations is what creates our life experience in every moment. Blair Singer in his book "Little Voice Mastery" states, "The reason many people never get to their dreams is that they are losing the ultimate 'little voice battle' being waged in their brains."

Did you just think, "What little voice? I don't have a little voice!" That's the one. We all have one. If you're like me and others I know, you probably have more than one.

Behavioral psychologists have proven that more than 77 percent of our self-talk is negative. Have you said to yourself, "Positive declarations or affirmations won't work for me for losing weight?" That's a declaration itself. Just thinking those words is a declaration. And, it has negative consequences. Your perception of being overweight can cause you to gain weight or prevent you from dropping it. Researchers found that thinking of yourself as being overweight can turn into a self-fulfilling prophecy.

According to a 2015 study in the *International Journal of Obesity*, individuals who considered themselves overweight were more likely to gain weight. The study also determined that telling an overweight person to lose weight isn't helpful because it could have a contrary effect. They found it caused more stress for the person, which contributed to that person maintaining their poor eating habits and patterns rather than changing. Remember, the number one reason people overeat and gain weight is because of stress.

Snack mixes, fries, cookies, M & Ms, and ice cream are go-to comfort foods because the high-carbs activate the brain's dopamine neuronal reward-motivated behavior. These foods act similarly to an addictive drug that makes you feel better. Again, it all comes down to mindset and how your mind affects your individual eating behavior.

Declarations and affirmations are important for weight loss because they work. Shad Helmstetter, Ph.D. is the author of more than 20 books in the field of personal growth, including *What to Say When You Talk to Yourself* and *Self-Talk for Weight Loss*. Dr. Helmstetter tells of a time when he was overweight and struggling with weight loss for many years. In his story he says he tried every diet imaginable and said all the wrong things to himself, thinking his weight problem would never go away. He says he would diet, lose weight, gain it all back, plus more. Then he'd try another diet and repeat the process.

Dr. Helmstetter said that during his struggles with weight he began to study self-talk. He learned that some professional athletes competing in the Olympics would hire full-time self-talk trainers to keep them motivated. He thought if Olympic athletes could have a full-time self-talk trainer to help them compete for gold medals, then what about the "Olympics of weight loss?" With that thought, an idea emerged.

He spent the next several months writing his own affirmations and declarations about his weight loss. Then he recorded them on audio. He'd listen to his affirmations and declarations in the

David Medansky

background while he shaved each morning. Morning after morning he'd repeat the process of listening to his voice state his affirmations and declarations.

During the next ten and one-half weeks he lost 38 pounds just shaving and playing his self-talk. And he wasn't on a diet. But another interesting and remarkable thing occurred. During the same ten and one-half weeks of intentionally listening to his own pep talk and losing weight, his wife was also dropping weight. She'd listen to his words while putting on her make-up while he shaved. She lost 25 pounds. That was more than 20 years ago, and he has never been on another diet since.

Unfortunately, most people engage in self-talk in a negative way. The types of affirmations people use are negative in nature. Do you use words and thoughts intended to build yourself up, or do you gravitate towards things keeping you down? Have you thought, *"Once I lose weight, I'll be good enough."*? Or, *"I'm too fat and ugly now, but when I lose weight, I'll have a boyfriend."* This is a Negative Motivation. While negative motivation can provide a short spurt of weight loss drive, it will ultimately not work out long term. Negative motivation may help you lose 20 to 30 pounds, but you'll likely be mentally worse off than before, and you may even regain the weight you've lost.

To successfully lose weight *and maintain healthy body weight for life*, you'll need to fix the negative self-talk you've been engaging in. The fix for this is simple. Here is how you can do it:

1. Identify the negative self-talk you've been using in your life (It might help to write these down so that you don't forget them).
2. Create positive affirmations around your negative self-talk. The goal here will be to literally "flip" your negative self-talk into positive affirmations.

Here are some examples:

"I am not overweight" becomes *"I am at my ideal weight."*

"I am losing weight" becomes *"I am closer and closer to my ideal weight with each and every day."*

"I am not eating junk food or fast food" becomes *"Everything I eat heals and nourishes my body which helps me reach my ideal weight."*

Get control over your thoughts, over your words and over yourself. It's going to require consistent work to reverse the psychological damage that negative self-talk causes within us. It won't happen overnight. But, give it enough time and the weight will melt off.

It's important to use the present tense when you create your new positive affirmations because the present tense will make them feel more sincere, authentic, and genuine. This will accelerate your progress. If you use the future tense such as one day or someday, it puts it off. Make it happen now. "I am..."

If you find yourself thinking or engaging in any negative self-talk - stop yourself. Transform it into the positive, right then and there. Focus on what you do want, not on what you don't want, because what you focus on expands. Here are suggested Weight-Reduction Daily Declarations. These are my personal declarations. You can choose which ones you want to adopt as yours or you can create your own.

1. I am in the process of being thin and fit.
2. I am in the process of making better food choices.
3. I choose to get rid of weight.
4. I am in the process of being worry free, stress-free, and drama free.
5. I am in the process of being an inspiration to others. If they have done it, I can do it. If I can do it, others can do it, so long as they have the want and desire to do so.
6. I act to reduce weight despite stress.
7. I act to reduce weight despite feeling hungry.
8. I avoid eating when I am stressed, nervous, anxious, or bored and find an alternative.
9. I am resolved to reducing weight in a healthy manner.
10. I encourage myself with positive self-talk.
11. I embrace the challenge of reducing weight. I understand it will not be easy.

12. I act despite what others might think or say.

13. I adopt the philosophy, "Your issues are not my issues."

14. My clothes tell me everything about being thinner.

Use "I Am" Statements

Affirmations are different from declarations. An affirmation states that a goal is already happening, whereas, a declaration is stating the objective of doing something. Staci Danford, a Gratitude Neuro Scientist, says you can achieve and maintain a healthy weight using *gratitude*. It must be sincere, and you must believe the words you say.

Below are suggested Healthy Weight Affirmations with *gratitude*. These are my personal "I am" statements. You can choose which ones you want to adopt as yours or you can create your own. Or, you can continue to use your declarations because they are similar.

- I am grateful, appreciative, and happy to be reducing weight.
- I am grateful and happy to be healthy and fit.
- I am grateful to be strong and beautiful at my healthy weight.
- I am grateful and happy retaining my healthy weight.
- I am grateful to be lighthearted. I attract joy and sincere, loving relationships.
- I am grateful I eat proper portions. I enjoy using a salad plate instead of a dinner plate.
- I am grateful to be an inspiration to others. If I can do it, others can too!
- I am grateful to be living a healthy lifestyle and improve each day.
- I am grateful my body is a fat-burning machine.
- I am grateful to be accountable for my choices.
- I am grateful to use great alternatives to keep focused and committed to my goals.
- I am grateful to be resolved to sustaining my reduced weight in a healthy manner.

- I am grateful to use positive words with myself and others.
- I am grateful my healthy eating habits make me smile with pride.
- I am grateful to allow myself to make food choices and decisions for my higher good regardless of what others might say or think.
- I am grateful to look and feel terrific. I love my body.

Let's recap. The simple elements to achieving and maintaining a healthy weight, according to Dr. David L. Katz, M.D., are:

- Eat holistic (whole) foods
- Mostly plants
- Not too much
- Avoid processed foods
- Drink lots of pure water
- The one additional element I added is to get adequate sleep.

The ten eating behaviors to change and improve are:

1. Drink more water
2. Avoid processed foods
3. Eat whole or holistic foods
4. Read and understand nutrition labels
5. Reduce portion sizes
6. Eat slower
7. Reduce or avoid alcoholic beverages
8. Watch your thoughts, watch your words -they have an impact
9. Stop eating at least three hours before going to sleep
10. Get adequate sleep

Create a personal Code of Honor for your weight-reduction journey; engage others to keep you accountable and provide you support; think in positive terms for weight reduction, and use declarations and affirmations with gratitude to reduce weight.

To be successful with anything you must be able to negotiate and communicate what it is you want. But, sometimes the toughest sale of all is selling yourself. It's like when you say to yourself, "I need to exercise today." Another voice in your head says, "No, I'm too tired." So, then you say to yourself, "I'll do it tomorrow." Or, "I'll do it after work."

Every person who has tried to lose weight knows that battle. It's the self-talk or management of it, that will get you through difficult times, or cause you to succumb. Don't let the negativity in, don't let your emotions even get started. Just tell yourself, "No thank you. I've practiced for this situation and I can control myself." Now you know what to do, and how to improve your eating behavior. The only question is, will you?

Stop being afraid of what can go wrong and start being positive about what could go right.

Chapter 6

Food Journal
It's More than Counting Calories

None of us is perfect.
But we can strive to improve each day.

In this chapter, you'll learn the importance of keeping a food journal for weight loss and how to properly keep track of your food intake. The most common reason people seem to keep food journals is for weight loss.

The four most common obstacles to keeping a food diary are:
- People are embarrassed or ashamed about what they eat.
- People have a sense of hopelessness, a feeling that it won't help to fill out a food diary.
- People feel it's too inconvenient to write down what they eat and drink.
- People feel bad or get upset with themselves when they "slip up."

What can you do to overcome these obstacles and challenges? By remembering a food journal is an effective tool to reduce weight. There is plenty of empirical evidence, based on research by several organizations, that keeping track of your daily food intake is one of the most effective ways you can change your eating behavior to reduce weight.

In 2009, a group of researchers funded by the National Institute of Health published a study for a different approach to losing weight. They asked 1,600 participants to write down everything they ate for at least one day per week. Notice I said one day per week – not every day.

After six months, those who kept a food log lost twice as much as those who didn't. The researchers learned that many participants started looking at their entries and finding patterns they didn't know existed.

Do you think you can keep track of everything you eat and drink for at least one day per week?

The participants started to implement different behavior modifications that were not suggested by the researchers. Some participants noticed they snacked at 10:00 a.m. so they started keeping an apple or banana in their desk for a midmorning snack instead of hitting the vending machine. Others started using their journals to plan future meals, such as dinner, so they could eat healthier rather than stop at the drive-thru for fast food or junk food in the fridge.

It's been proven that keeping track of what you eat is the most effective method for controlling and reducing your daily caloric, carbs, fat, sugar, and protein intake. Whether you call it a daily food diary, diet journal, calorie tracker, food journal, or diet log, keeping track of your food intake is all about accountability. It's not what you do when someone is watching, it's what you do when no one is watching. Be honest with yourself. Keep your integrity. Tell the truth. Note it in your log if you indulged and ate the slice of birthday cake at the office party. No one is judging you.

According to a study by Kaiser Permanente's Center for Health Research in 2008, keeping a food diary can double a person's weight loss. Their findings were published in the August 2008 issue (Volume 35, Issue 2, Pages 118–126) of *American Journal of Preventive Medicine*. Jack Hollis Ph.D., a researcher at Kaiser Permanente's Center for Health Research, said, "The more food records people kept, the more weight they lost. Those who kept daily food records lost twice as much weight as those who kept no records. It seems that the simple act of writing down what you eat encourages people to consume fewer calories."

The Kaiser Permanente's study was conducted in four cities, Portland, Oregon; Baltimore, Maryland; Durham, North Carolina, and Baton Rouge, Louisiana. In involved 1,685 middle-aged men and women over six months. The average age of the participants in the study was 55.

Food journaling isn't easy or convenient but done consistently, it can help you move to more healthful choices. It allows you to keep track of calories, and other aspects of your dietary behaviors and habits. Keeping a food diary/log/record is an important tool in dietary self-awareness, and one of the best ways to improve your eating habits. You can use anything to record your food intake, such as printed booklets, low-tech notebooks, ready-made apps on iPhones, smartphones, or tablets. Use whatever works best for you.

Kerri Anne Hawkins, a dietitian with Tufts Medical Center's Obesity Consultation Center, uses several types of food diary forms for her patients. She tells them to fill out just what works for them; they can even create their own system, like using sticky notes.

Let's discuss some basic information to keep track of to guide you. Because it's not just about calories. On the food logs we use, there is an area to keep track of how many glasses of water you drink in a day. Remember, over 75 percent of Americans suffer from chronic dehydration. Having an area to keep track of drinking Apple Cider Vinegar and

Lemon Juice is important. Why?

Because Apple Cider Vinegar and lemon juice have many health benefits. Some of these benefits include:

- Apple Cider Vinegar Helps Body Reduce Fat
- Apple Cider Vinegar Improves Digestion
- Apple Cider Vinegar Balances pH Levels
- Apple Cider Vinegar Maintains Blood Sugar Levels
- Apple Cider Vinegar promotes Detoxification of Liver

Studies have shown Apple Cider Vinegar:

- Increases Metabolism
- Suppresses the Appetite
- Helps in Oxidation of Stored Fat
- Contains Pectin, a naturally occurring soluble fiber
- It's Rich in Calcium & Potassium – which promote weight loss

By itself, Apple Cider Vinegar does not cause weight loss. But, in conjunction with reducing calories, increased water intake, and improved eating habits, it can help you lose weight. But it will only provide results if used consistently over a prolonged time. Be patient.

NOTE: Never drink undiluted apple cider vinegar. Apple cider vinegar should be consumed in water or another liquid because the acid can ruin teeth enamel.

Apple cider vinegar can be used as a salad dressing by mixing 1/2 to 1 teaspoon with 1 tablespoon of extra virgin olive oil and 1 to 2 tablespoons of lemon juice. (Maybe add some ground black pepper and garlic powder.)

The benefits of Lemon Juice include:
- Promotes hydration
- Good source of vitamin C
- Supports weight loss
- Aids digestion
- Prevents kidney stones

Mix one tablespoon of apple cider vinegar and one tablespoon of lemon juice in eight ounces of pure water in the morning. There is an area on the food log to indicate that this was done.

It's also important to keep track of your sugar intake, how many carbohydrates you eat, and whether they are simple carbs or complex carbs. Contrary to some fad diets, not all carbs are bad. Good carbs are required and necessary for proper nutrition and food balance.

You'll also need to note if you're getting enough protein and fiber. It's important to make sure you're getting enough protein and fiber each day. Most people do not get enough, yet think they do.

What about fats? Are you eating enough healthy good fats and avoiding the bad and scientifically engineered fats?

We shall see.

Be thorough. Note whether the food was fried or broiled; include all toppings, sauces, and condiments. Note all beverages, including cream, sugar, and flavored syrup. And always remember to keep track of portions.

Calories: To lose a pound each week, you must reduce your intake by about 500 calories per day. For example, if you normally eat 2,000 calories per day, to lose weight you must eat closer to 1,500 calories per day. It is recommended you reduce your calories so that you're eating between 1,250 and 1,500 per day. Reduce your caloric intake gradually.

Here's an example. If you're used to consuming 3,000 or more calories per day, give yourself time to adjust. Again, the goal is to reduce your caloric intake by 500 calories per day until you are comfortable eating less. Counting calories may have a negative impact on you losing weight. The reason being that people tend to overestimate how many calories they burn and underestimate how many calories they consume. Further, low-calorie recipes in several magazines looked delicious, but reading the fine print can be alarming.

Many of these low-calorie dishes were loaded with a lot of sodium, ranging between 450 to 1,000 mg or more per serving; high carbohydrates, ranging between 35 to 69 grams or more per serving.

There are benefits to monitoring your food intake in other ways than just counting calories.

As you will recall, it's important to get adequate sleep. Because the average person, when sleep deprived, will consume an extra 500 per day. And to lose one pound you must reduce your caloric intake by 500 calories per day for an entire week.

Can you relate to eating more when you're tired?

Grams of Protein: You should eat between four and seven ounces of lean protein at each meal. There are about 7 grams of protein in 1 ounce of cooked meat. Eating enough protein is important to losing weight because it's well-supported by science that protein can boost a person's metabolic rate and curb the appetite.

Studies done on protein, as it relates to weight loss, indicate that consuming 25 to 30 percent protein as a percentage of your total daily calories can boost your metabolism by up to 80 to 100 calories per day, compared to lower protein diets.

Protein also can reduce your appetite because it keeps you feeling fuller compared to both fat and carbs. A study done about obese men reported in *Obesity (Silver Springs)* April 19, 2011, issue showed that protein at 25 percent of daily calories increased feelings of fullness, reduced the desire for late-night snacking by half and reduced obsessive thoughts about food by 60 percent.

In another study reported in the *American Journal of Clinical Nutrition*, July 2005, women who increased their protein intake to 30 percent of their daily calories ate 441 fewer calories per day. The women lost 11 pounds in 12 weeks simply by adding more protein to their diet.

It's been found that protein not only helps you lose weight, but it can also prevent you from gaining weight in the first place. In one study reported in the *International Journal of Obesity and Related Metabolic Disorders*, January 2004 issue, a modest increase in protein from 15 percent to 18 percent of calories reduced the amount of fat people regained after weight loss by 50 percent.

According to these and other studies, a protein intake of around 30 percent of calories seems to be optimal for weight loss. This amounts to 150 grams per day for someone on a 2,000- calorie diet. You can calculate how much protein as a percentage of your daily caloric intake by multiplying your calorie intake by 0.075. As an example, if you're consuming 1,500 calories per day, your protein intake should be about 112 grams.

Fried chicken or fried fish does not count as a good source of protein because the oil used to fry the food offsets and benefits. Baked, grilled, or broiled chicken, fish, or meat is the best.

No, a hot dog or bratwurst does not count as a good protein. Again, they are processed foods with too much sodium and nitrates to be beneficial to your weight-reduction endeavors.

Carbohydrates: Keep your carbohydrate intake between 20 and 50 grams per day. Keep in mind there is a difference between complex carbohydrates as opposed to simple carbohydrates. Avoid simple carbs.

Examples of simple carbohydrates include, but are not limited to, rice, potatoes, pasta, bread, anything made from grains, bagels, refined sugar, peas, corn, jams, and jellies, etc. Note: Although beans and lentils are complex carbohydrates, you should limit the amount you consume because they contain a lot of starch.

Fat: Between 40 and 53 grams of healthy fat per day is suggested to reduce weight. There are good fats, bad fats, and ugly fats. The good fats are unsaturated fats. Unsaturated fats include polyunsaturated fatty acids and monounsaturated fats. The bad fats are saturated fats and trans fats (partially hydrogenated fats). And avoid the scientifically engineered fat substitutes such as Olean.

Sugar: Refined sugar should be avoided. There is no daily requirement for added sugars. Refined sugar doesn't serve any physiological purpose. The less you eat, the healthier you will be. Refined sugar is addicting. Be wary of Starbucks and other specialty shops with trendy or indulgent coffee drinks. Many of their flavored drinks have as much as 71 grams of sugar. According to the American Heart Association, your body needs less than 36 grams of added sugar per day for men and 24 grams for women. A 12 ounce can of Coke has 39 grams of sugar. A 1.55-ounce Hershey's chocolate bar has 24 grams of sugar.

Imagine how many people have a can of Coke and a Hershey bar from the vending machines for a mid-afternoon snack. In other words, you are getting more sugar (refined sugar at that) in one snack than you need for an entire day.

Can you relate to this?

And we wonder why more than 70 percent of the American population is overweight.

Fiber: Aim for at least 38 grams of fiber per day if you're a male under age 50 and 25 grams if you're a female under age 50 (or 21 and 30 grams daily, respectively, for those over the age of 50). Are you getting enough fiber each day? Are you sure? If you aren't certain you're getting enough dietary fiber each day, track your food intake for a few days or a week.

Fiber is important to reduce constipation. Constipation is a silent epidemic because most people do not want to talk about. Going to the bathroom is a private matter. I'm even uncomfortable talking about this topic.

For many people, constipation is little more than an aggravation. To others, it is a daily agony. Few realize that it can be a dangerous and even deadly affliction. But, in 2016, constipation was the reason for six million doctors' visits and 700,000 emergency room visits. This cost billions of dollars in health care costs, along with what Americans spend on over-the-counter laxatives. Chronic constipation can be avoided by changing and improving your eating habits.

Eating a diet with low fiber and lack of enough water causes people to use medications such as laxatives and enemas that can have a negative effect on your bowels.

Can you relate to this issue?

The number of people admitted to the hospital primarily for constipation has more than doubled since 1997.

So, how can you get more fiber in your diet? Here are some suggestions. An avocado has 10 grams of fiber. An apple has 4.4 grams. Those two items alone have 14.4 grams. More than one-third of what you need for a day if you're a man and more than half if you're a woman.

What else should you include in your food log? Rebecca Puhl, Ph.D., director of research at the Rudd Center for Food Policy and Obesity at Yale University, suggests including the location of the meal because these details will provide insight into emotional triggers for eating habits and places where you are most likely to consume healthy and unhealthy foods.

If you're trying to understand how your emotions relate to your food choices, you might also want to include questions in your diary such as, "How hungry am I?" or "What were my emotions before, during, and after the eating episode?"

You should log the details of your food consumption as you go throughout the day or set some time aside at the end of the day to update it. But experts say your record will be more accurate if you do it right after eating. They also say it's important to record everything – even if that seems painful.

While writing in your food journal every day is best, it is not necessary. If possible, write in your food diary for at least five days each week. Remember at the beginning of this chapter you were told that people who recorded everything they ate just one day per week had significant results. Do what will work best for you so long as what you're doing is producing positive results.

And, while it can be tempting to not record a binge episode or eating an impromptu dessert, this is the most important time to track it.

Be certain to log in what you ate, why, where, and how much. The reason being it can provide you with valuable insight that can help you change and improve your eating habits.

If you just can't bring yourself to fill out a detailed food diary form each day, that's OK. Just writing a minimum amount of information in your food diary will help you in your weight-loss journey. Many people believe that it's necessary to keep a "perfect" food log with every detail, and if they don't, they have failed. It is not necessary or required to keep a perfect food log. Your efforts to record what you eat and drink gets you closer to paying attention to your food choices and habits.

Be motivated and inspired on your weight reduction journey. In addition to the tracking of your food each day, this journal is designed to help you see the connections between your emotions and what you eat, why you eat, when you eat, and the reason you eat. A simple journal should provide enough information to allow you to see trends that may be causing your weight to stall or gain, an awareness which can ultimately help you accomplish your incremental weight-reduction goals and increase your total weight-reduction.

Fill in the journal every day if possible because this will show your connection between food and moods as well as general eating patterns. The more information you fill in, the more patterns you'll see. Change your attitude and your body as you read each declaration or affirmation you learned in the previous lesson.

If you work with a counselor, doctor, or dietician (or are planning to), share your journal with them.

If you find yourself wanting to journal everything you eat in detail, don't. It is not something you should do for the rest of your life. To help you curb the impulse to meticulously chart everything you eat, only a small space is provided on the food journal in Appendix E. This gives you enough space to record your meals and snacks in case you run into problems but prevents you from spending too much time on it.

You'll notice that some food journals have three meals: Breakfast, Lunch, and Dinner, plus three snacks: Mid-morning, mid-afternoon, and after dinner. If you can control your food consumption to these specific times, you should see positive results. If possible, avoid eating after 7:00 p.m. If not, try to eat your last bit of food at least three hours before you go to sleep.

It's simple: three meals, three snacks throughout the day.

Note – If you're not able to have a snack or miss a snack, don't worry about it or try to make it up. Not everyone needs to eat constantly throughout the day.

Drink at least eight 8 ounces glasses of pure water each day. My preference is to drink distilled water. There are arguments on both sides whether this is good or bad. You make your own decision. Pure water is better for you than sodas, flavored water, carbonated water, or fruit juices.

Avoid Orange juice and other fruit juices. Fruit juices have too much fructose, glucose, and sucrose. As an example, would you ever sit down and eat four oranges? One orange is plenty. But it takes four medium oranges to make an 8 ounces glass of orange juice. Juicing removes the fiber and gives you 28 grams of carbohydrates.

Questions to keep in mind as you complete the food journal:
- Are certain foods causing mood swings?
- Do you use food to improve your mood or energy?
- Are there certain times of the day or situations when you're susceptible to cravings?
- Out of habit do you associate certain activities with eating, such as watching TV, eating popcorn at a movie theater, etc?
- Does an increased level of stress cause you to eat more?
- What types of food do you crave?
- Is too much caffeine causing anxiety or mood swings?

Food for Thought - Things to Ponder and Contemplate to Gain Insight Into Your Eating Habits

Dr. Joseph Mercola, in his book, *Fat for Food Ketogenic Cookbook,* stated, "…when Hippocrates wrote, 'Let food be thy medicine and medicine be thy food,' he shared an elemental truth: if your food isn't contributing to your health, it's contributing to your illness."

Note the time and location, and your mood and satiety, to help you identify patterns and triggers. Why are you eating a mid-afternoon bag of chips? How much of your caloric intake occurs while you are watching TV?

Time: Writing down when you eat helps you to see if emotional eating happens at specific times. Is your eating hunger-driven or is it because you're emotional?

If possible, the best time to eat your meals is between 7:00 a.m. and 7:00 p.m. Some advocate for a smaller window to consume your food. But, with a 12-hour period, it gives your body 12 hours to process and digest your food.

Why Are You Eating?

Are you stressed? Anxious? Upset about something or someone? Do you eat when you're nervous? Are you eating when you're lonely or sad? Do you eat when you're bored? Are you eating for comfort? Or, are you consuming food as fuel for your body? Emotional eating can be modified and altered once you're aware that it's happening.

Here are the reasons people gave as to why they ate:

- I ate when I was bored.
- I ate when I'd watch television.
- I ate when I was worried or stressed.
- I ate when I was frustrated or upset.
- I ate to reward myself.
- I ate to make myself feel better.
- I ate because I was lonely.

You might be able to add a few reasons of your own.

Did you notice what all the reasons have in common?

Give up?

Not one reason given for eating was for nutrition or for fuel for your body.

All animals in their natural state, except for humans, eat *only* for the purpose of maintaining health and nutrition. Humans are the only species that eats for pleasure and comfort.

According to Dr. Shad Helmstetter, "We overeat to fulfill the needs of the mind."

The reason you should eat is for nutrition and as fuel for your body. Keep this in mind when you are recording what you are eating. Because it's just as important to understand why you are eating as what you're eating. Once you understand that eating should be to provide fuel and proper nourishment for your body, you'll have a different perspective about food.

Can you see how your perception of food could change and improve your eating habits?

What Type of Food Are You Eating?

Writing down what you eat helps you see connections between moods and certain foods. Are you tempted to eat cookies or ice cream when you're stressed? Or, do reach for a candy bar when you're nervous? Or, maybe you prefer salty foods such as potato chips, pretzels, or something crunchy if you're lonely or feeling sad? Are you eating foods that satiate you or just lead to more cravings? Are you getting any protein?

Environment: Does what's happening around you affect your eating? Some people tend to snack when watching TV; others turn to food if other family members are eating too. Where are you eating? At the kitchen table? While watching TV? In your car driving? At your desk in your office or at work? A restaurant? Does where you eat increase the quantity you consume? If so, you might consider consciously changing the location of your meals.

Watching television detrimentally affects your eating habits which can cause obesity. Studies show a direct correlation between watching television and weight gain. People tend to snack on calorie-dense processed foods while viewing the boob tube. Studies have shown that viewers consume 65 percent more calories from snacks while watching television.

Have you noticed that commercials displayed on the screen during prime time and late at night are prominently for food and restaurants? They're designed and created to entice you to eat more. Further, eating late at night is the worst time to chow down. To add insult to injury, the advertisements usually depict thin people. If you have a poor self-image you might consume more food to comfort yourself. Television commercials provide conflicting, confusing, and misleading information about proper nutrition. Because of this, people who watch a lot of television tend to have a poorer understanding of healthy eating. "This Bud's for you. Dilly, Dilly."

One study found 34 percent of viewers were more likely to order high-fat, high-sugar foods from menus than those who didn't watch television. Who wants to order a pizza from Pizza Hut, Little Caesars, or Dominoes? Perhaps by keeping a food journal, you'll discover you're watching a lot more television than you thought.

What can you do to combat a television eating habit?

Do a few push-ups in between commercials. The average commercial break is between two to five minutes. Instead of getting up to grab a snack, do some push-ups. Even if you start with five. You can build up to doing 25 to 50 push-ups during a commercial break. Do some leg lifts. Again, start slowly and build up. Before you know it, you'll be doing 25 to 50 leg lifts during each commercial break along with your push-ups.

Not fond of leg lifts? Do squats. Or, grab light-weight dumbbells. There are many things you can do during a commercial break to get some physical activity. Imagine, you won't need to go to the gym to do a workout. You'll save time and money.

The average one-hour long television show has between seven and 10 commercial breaks. If you can build up to doing just 25 push-ups during just four commercial interruptions, you'd have done 100 push-ups. Do it gradually if you haven't done much or any exercise in a while.

You might consider tracking how many hours you spend watching television. It may surprise you how much time you're wasting in front of the screen.

Do you watch television in your bedroom? This can disrupt sleep and cause other health issues. Research shows that the nighttime glow streaming from the television throws off biorhythms, messes with hunger signals, and has a direct correlation to weight gain. A simple solution is to remove the culprit from the bedroom or make certain it is off before you go to sleep.

Track your eating behavior for a few weeks. Then look for patterns. If it appears there's a relationship between eating and feelings, think of ways to meet the emotional needs without turning to food. Ask people in the support community for suggestions. Or, if they will be an accountability buddy you can talk to avoid comfort eating. Maybe take a walk, do some yoga or quick exercise. Find other ways to deal with frustration.

Starting a food journal is one thing. Sticking with it is another matter and ideally, it's something that should be done for weeks rather than days. "Food journaling is hard," said James Fogarty, associate professor of computer science and engineering at the University of Washington, in Seattle. The medical literature talks about non-compliance and that many people will only record in a journal for a few days or only a week and give up. Dr. Fogarty and co-researchers have explored the barriers to keeping a food journal by examining several online food journal websites to see how design might influence the difficulty people often find sticking with them.

Write out what you plan to eat before eating it. This can sometimes be a deterrent to overeating or eating the wrong foods. You don't necessarily need to keep a journal for recording and tracking your food. Here's a little advice from Jim Rohn on keeping a journal for the past 40 plus years:

- "Be a collector of good ideas, but don't trust your memory. The best collecting place for all of the ideas and information that comes your way is your journal."
- "The reason why I spend so much money for my journals is to press me to find something valuable to put in them."
- "Don't use your mind for a filing cabinet. Use your mind to work out problems and find answers; file away good ideas in your journal."

Chapter 7

Reading and Understanding Nutrition Facts Labels

Change your habits, change your life.
Thomas C. Corley

Capital One Financial promotes its credit card services by asking "What's in your wallet?" William Devane in his commercials for Rosland Capital gold and silver asks, "What's in your safe?" Perhaps the better question to ask yourself is, "What's in your food?"

Do you read the nutritional labels on the cans, packages, or boxes of the food you purchase? If you do, do you understand what you're eating?

Do you read the fine print of those delicious low-calorie recipes in magazines? My guess is that you probably don't because most people won't.

In this chapter, you'll learn how to read and understand the information provided on the Nutrition Fact label required on all food packaging and the importance of reading the fine print in magazines that provide you with so-called healthy recipes.

Every packaged, or processed, product should have a label. Some restaurants also have nutrition information available. The Nutritional Fact label is also known as the Nutrition Facts panel. It was first introduced in 1993. The Food and Drug Administration updated the food labeling requirements in 2016 to make it easier to see how many calories and added sugars are in a product and to make serving sizes more realistic. The new requirements do not take effect until January 1, 2021. For now, you may see the redesigned version or an old version on a product.

The information shown in the Nutrition Facts label is based on a diet of 2,000 calories a day. You need less than 2,000 calories to reduce weight. Your daily caloric intake should be between 1,250 and 1,500.

Nutrition Facts

Serving Size 1 cup (228g)
Servings Per Container 2

(1) **Start Here** ➡

Amount Per Serving

(2) **Check Calories** | **Calories** 250   Calories from Fat 110

	% Daily Value* (6)
Total Fat 12g	**18%**
Saturated Fat 3g	**15%**
Trans Fat 3g	
Cholesterol 30mg	**10%**
Sodium 470mg	**20%**
Total Carbohydrate 31g	**10%**

(3) **Limit these Nutrients**

Quick Guide to % DV

Dietary Fiber 0g	**0%**
Sugars 5g	
Protein 5g	
Vitamin A	**4%**
Vitamin C	**2%**
Calcium	**20%**
Iron	**4%**

• **5% or less is Low**

• **20% or more is High**

(4) **Get Enough of these Nutrients**

(5) **Footnote**

* Percent Daily Values are based on a 2,000 calorie diet. Your Daily Values may be higher or lower depending on your calorie needs.

	Calories:	2,000	2,500
Total Fat	Less than	65g	80g
Sat Fat	Less than	20g	25g
Cholesterol	Less than	300mg	300mg
Sodium	Less than	2,400mg	2,400mg
Total Carbohydrate		300g	375g
Dietary Fiber		25g	30g

How to read and interpret the Nutrition Facts label will be broken down into five steps.

Step One: Start with the serving information at the top. The first place to start when you look at the Nutrition Facts label is the serving size and the number of servings in the package. Serving sizes are standardized to make it easier to compare similar foods; they are provided in familiar units, such as cups or pieces, followed by the metric amount, such as the number of grams.

The size of the serving on the food package influences the number of calories and all the nutrient amounts listed on the top part of the label. There is a difference between a serving size and a portion. A portion is the amount of food you choose to eat for a meal. Pay attention to the serving size, especially how many servings there are in the food package. Then ask yourself, "How many servings am I consuming?" For example, a standard 4-ounce can of tuna has two servings. If you eat the entire can of tuna your portion was two serving sizes. That doubles the calories and other nutrient numbers. Instead of 50 calories, you'd consume 100. Your sodium intake would be 180 mg instead of 90.

Step Two: Look at the total calories per serving. Calories provide a measure of how much energy you get from a serving of this food. Many Americans consume more calories than they need without meeting recommended intakes for several essential nutrients. Remember: Your portion amount is based on the number of servings you consume and that will determine the number of calories you eat. As a General Guide to Calories,

1. 40 calories is low
2. 100 calories is moderate
3. 400 calories or more is high

Eating too many calories per day is linked to being overweight and obese.

Step Three: The Nutrients. Some of the nutrients listed on a label are good while others are bad. The good nutrients include:

- **Fiber.** Fiber helps your body digest the food you eat. It also can help lower your risk of Type 2 diabetes and heart disease. Food is high in fiber if it contains 5 grams or more per serving. Men 50 years of age or younger should get at least 38 grams of fiber per day. Women 50 years of age or younger should get at least 25 grams of fiber per day. Fiber is found in fruits, vegetables, and whole grains. Look for the words "whole grain" on the package and ingredient list versus "multigrain." The multi grain is *not* the same as whole grain.

- **Vitamins and minerals.** The main types include vitamin A, vitamin C, calcium, and iron. Vitamin D and potassium also are important. Talk to your doctor about what vitamins and minerals you need and how much.
- **Fats.** Eating healthy fat is good for your body and will help you to stay satisfied throughout the day. Make sure you're aware of the difference between healthy fats and unhealthy fats. Polyunsaturated and monosaturated promote good health. We'll talk about the bad fats in a moment.
- **Protein.** Protein is important for maintaining muscle mass. When you select foods at the grocery store, read Nutrition Facts labels to choose foods that provide protein. However, the percentage of daily value for protein is not required on the label. Eat moderate portions of lean meat, poultry, fish, eggs, low-fat milk, yogurt, and cheese, plus beans and peas, peanut butter, and seeds.
- But when you check the nutrition label for protein, scan the fat grams to make sure the number is not too high. Many protein-rich foods are also high in saturated fat and some foods in the dairy and bakery aisles contain unhealthy trans fat. Nutrients that are bad for you and which you should avoid or eat less include:
  - Fat
  - Sodium
  - Carbohydrates
  - Sugars
- **Saturated fat is an unhealthy fat.** This type of fat can increase your risk of heart disease and high cholesterol. The average adult should consume less than 20 grams of saturated fat per day.
- **Trans fat.** This fat also increases your risk of heart disease. Experts could not provide a reference value

for trans fat nor any other information that the FDA believes adequate to establish a daily value or %DV.

Scientific reports link trans fat (and saturated fat) with raising blood LDL ("bad") cholesterol levels, both of which increase your risk of coronary heart disease, a leading cause of death in the U.S. Ideally, you should get 0 grams of trans fat per day. Companies can list 0 grams if it contains less than 0.5 grams of trans fat per serving. This means that your food may have trans fat even if the nutrition label says 0.

Check the ingredient list for trans fat products. This includes any partially hydrogenated oil and hydrogenated vegetable oils. Trans fat often is found in baked goods, fried foods, snack foods, and margarine. If you eat more than one serving, you could be eating too much trans fat.

- **Cholesterol.** You should eat less than 300 milligrams of cholesterol per day. If you have heart disease, aim for less than 200 milligrams per day.
- **Carbohydrates.** Whether or not you're counting carbs, choosing better sources of carbohydrates is important for good health.
- **Sugars**. It's smart to monitor your sugar intake for weight loss and maintenance, as well as overall good health. Selecting foods with a lower number is a good idea. The new Nutrition Facts panel makes it easier to choose healthier options by breaking out the amount of added sugar under the "Total Sugar" heading. Foods with more added sugars provide empty calories and provide very little nutrition. Select foods with fewer added sugars.

  Also, check the ingredients to make sure there are no ingredients ending in "OSE" or contain Aspartame and other artificial sweeteners. Simple carbohydrates, or sugars, occur naturally in foods such as fruit (fructose) and milk (lactose) or come from refined sources such as table sugar (sucrose) or corn syrup. Added sugars must be included on the Nutrition Facts label starting in 2018.

The 2015-2020 *Dietary Guidelines for Americans* recommends consuming no more than 10 percent of daily calories from added sugars.

- **Sodium**, or salt, is one nutrient that gets its own bolded line on the label because too much can be harmful to your health. Most experts recommend that healthy adults limit their sodium intake to no more than 2,300 milligrams per day. If you have a specific health condition, such as high blood pressure or kidney disease, consult your doctor or nutritionist to determine the right amount for you. Low sodium amounts to 140 milligrams or less per serving.

Step Four: Percent of Daily Value. The numbers listed under "% Daily Value" tell you how much a specific nutrient contributes to your total daily diet if you consume 2,000 calories per day. If you consume more or less than 2,000 calories per day, these percentages will not be accurate for you, but they are still useful in making healthy food choices.

Overall, the % Daily Value can quickly help you gauge whether a food is high or low in a nutrient. Generally, a daily value of 5 percent or less means that the food is low in that nutrient and a value of 20 percent or more means that the food is high in the nutrient.

Use the % Daily Value numbers to help evaluate how a food fits into your daily meal plan. Remember, %Daily Value covers the entire day, not just one meal or snack. A food serving with a 5 percent Daily Value of fat provides 5 percent of the total fat that a person consuming 2,000 calories a day should eat.

You may need more or less than 2,000 calories per day. For some nutrients, you may need more or less than 100 percent Daily Value.

Low is 5 percent or less. Aim low in saturated fat, trans fat, cholesterol, and sodium.

High is 20 percent or more. Aim high in vitamins, minerals, and fiber.

To summarize: The % Daily Value tells you the percentage of each nutrient in a single serving, in terms of the daily recommended amount for a 2,000 calorie a day diet. If you want to consume less of a nutrient (such as saturated fat or sodium), choose foods with a lower % Daily Value (5 percent or less). If you want to consume more of a nutrient (such as fiber), choose foods with a higher % DV (20 percent or more).

Step Five: Source of Fiber.

- **Dietary fiber.** Fiber is good for you. You'll feel full longer if you eat foods with more dietary fiber. Plus, selecting foods with a higher amount of dietary fiber may help you stick with your new and improved eating behavior. Packaged foods that contain whole grains or vegetables like spinach are often good sources of dietary fiber. Some foods also provide added fiber which may be helpful for some healthy eaters.

Eating a diet high in dietary fiber promotes healthy bowel function. Additionally, a diet rich in fruits, vegetables, and grain products that contain dietary fiber, particularly soluble fiber, and low in saturated fat and cholesterol may reduce the risk of heart disease.

Consider the additional nutrients listed on the label. You know about calories, but it also is important to know about the other nutrients on the Nutrition Facts label. Make sure you get enough of the nutrients your body needs, such as calcium, choline, dietary fiber, iron, magnesium, potassium, and vitamins A, C, D, and E.*

Note the * used after the heading "%Daily Value" on the Nutrition Facts label. It refers to the Footnote in the lower part of the nutrition label, which tells you "%DVs are based on a 2,000-calorie diet." This statement must be on all food labels. But the remaining information in the full footnote may not be on the package if the size of the label is too small. When the full footnote does appear, it will always be the same. It doesn't change from product to product, because it shows recommended dietary advice for all Americans--it is not about a specific food product.

READ THE INGREDIENTS!

According to Vani Hari, *The Food Babe*, New York Times bestselling author of *The Food Babe Way: Break Free from the*

Hidden Contaminants in Your Food and Lose Weight, Look Years Younger, and Get Healthy in Just 21 Days! and *Feeding You Lies: How to Unravel the Food Industry's Playbook and Reclaim Your Health* suggests you ask yourself these three questions before eating: 1) What are the ingredients? 2) Are the ingredients nutritious? 3) Where do the ingredients come from?

If you are concerned about your intake of sugars, make sure that added sugars are not listed as one of the first few ingredients. Other names for added sugars include corn syrup, high-fructose corn syrup, fruit juice concentrate, maltose, dextrose, sucrose, honey, and maple syrup.

Foods with more than one ingredient must have an ingredient list on the label. Ingredients are listed in descending order by weight. Those in the largest amounts are listed first. This information is particularly helpful to individuals with food sensitivities, those who wish to avoid pork or shellfish, limit added sugars or people who prefer vegetarian eating.

Learn how to read nutrition labels before deciding whether to eat the food or not.

My best advice to you is to eat real food. An avocado or apple will provide you with more nutritional benefits than processed products.

Chapter 8

Goals

Well done is better than well said.
Benjamin Franklin

Do you have written goals?

In this chapter, you'll learn the importance of setting goals for reducing weight.

It is vital to understand that getting rid of weight is a process. There is no instantaneous solution to sustainable weight reduction. Achieving a healthy weight and maintaining it requires long-term changes to the way you think and feel about food. View food as fuel for your body. Stop putting CRAP into your body. CRAP stands for:

C = carbonated drinks

R = refined sugars

A = artificial foods

P = process foods

You are what you eat, so don't be fast, cheap, easy, or fake.

Goals help you define what you really want: reducing weight, getting thinner, becoming healthier, or all of these. You must set specific, realistic, and attainable goals that can be accomplished in a timely manner. Some refer to this as S.M.A.R.T. goals. Your ambition to lose as much weight as possible is neither specific or realistic. Saying, "I want to lose weight" or "I want to exercise more" are broad, vague statements.

Do you go to Las Vegas? You're probably wondering what does Las Vegas have to do with reducing weight? Absolutely nothing.

But it has a lot to do with illustrating the importance of setting specific, realistic, and attainable goals. Some people who go to Vegas have the attitude, "I want to win as much as possible." What does that mean? Does it mean you want to win $500 or $5,000 or more? It's not specific.

Others will have the mindset, "I'll take $100 and stop once I lose it." To me, that's a defeatist mentality.

When I go to Vegas my goal is to win 20 percent of my buy-in for each session I play. So, if I buy-in for $500, my goal is to win $100 for the session. That is specific and realistic.

Are you starting to understand? If I ask you, "Would you like to weigh 20, 30, or 40 pounds lighter by this time next year?" you'd probably nod your head. Would you agree that you could probably lose two, three, or four pounds in a month? That's doable. If you did lose two, three, or four pounds each month for 12 consecutive months, after one year you'd have accomplished weighing 20 to 40 pounds less.

To be more specific with your weight-reduction goal, you might aim to lose one or two pounds per week. If you think losing one or two pounds per week is too small of an amount, you might be surprised that it is not. Because if you did lose one to two pounds per week for four consecutive weeks, you'd have lost four to eight pounds in a month. If you did that for 12 consecutive months, that would be 48 to 96 pounds in a year. So, losing one to two pounds per week is no small accomplishment as long as it is done consistently over a long period of time. Even if you cut that in half, you'd still shed between 24 and 48 pounds in a year.

Remember, simply making small adjustments to your daily eating behaviors consistently over a long period of time (like a year) will give you noticeable results. Think of it this way, making small adjustments to your daily eating behaviors to lose one to two pounds per week, done consistently for 52 weeks will result in a total weight loss of between 52 pounds and 104 pounds during a year. Now you might not be able to consistently shed one to two pounds per week because as you get lighter, your body needs to adjust to the lower weight and may plateau. But, if you can average three to four pounds per month for 12 consecutive months, that would be 36 to 48 pounds in a year.

For most, it took over five, ten, or 15 years to accumulate your extra weight. If you have a burning desire to reduce weight in a healthy and sustainable fashion, your body can accomplish an amazing transformation. A goal is a road map that provides an explicit idea of what you want to be and a plan of action to get there. W. Edward Deming said, "A goal without a method is nonsense." Make certain you have a method to achieve your weight-reduction goal. A motivational meme said, "A goal without a plan is just a wish." Individuals who have successful weight-reduction regimens take the time to create a clear plan. Attempting to reduce weight without a plan is like going from A to Z without stopping in between.

Have you set a goal but did not have a plan to accomplish it?

The fact is that you've been given a plan to reduce weight in prior chapters. You learned how to change and improve 10 eating behaviors over 10 months that will give you a lifetime of results for achieving and maintaining a healthy weight. Have of you started to implement what you learned yet?

Every life coach or personal trainer knows the importance of goals. They give something an aim to achieve and a way to measure it. For weight-reduction there are two ways to measure your success: 1) the dreaded scale or 2) your clothes to tell you how you're doing.

The simple process to reduce weight is 1) decide to commit to reducing weight, 2) plan how you're going to achieve it (albeit you have been given 10 eating behaviors to modify and improve during the next 10 months), and 3) measure your results along the way.

Decide your total desired weight-reduction goal and work toward achieving it in increments. People who are successful in reducing weight are very clear about their intentions. Those who fail are generally vague or uncertain. For example, if you decide to reduce your overall weight by 35 pounds, set a target to lose three pounds each month for 12 consecutive months. Achieving smaller objectives does three things:

1. Provides a systematic process
2. Creates a sense of accomplishment
3. Gives you small victories to celebrate

Achieving results, no matter how small, helps to keep you on course and encouraged to stay motivated to shed weight.

How do you eat an elephant? One bite at a time.

How did you gain your weight? One bite at a time.

How will you reduce weight in a healthy and sustainable manner? One pound at a time.

Start small and create a win for yourself. When you do this, you build confidence. With confidence, you gain momentum. With momentum, you take more action to move closer to your goal. Nothing sustains motivation more than a sense of accomplishment. Another motivational quote about goals stated, and I'm paraphrasing to remove the vulgar language, "Set goals, stay quiet about them, smash them, clap for yourself, repeat." That's a nice quote, but it still does not provide a plan to accomplish your goal. Perhaps it should state, "Set goals, plan how to accomplish them, keep them to yourself, accomplish them, celebrate and repeat."

Let's talk about S.M.A.R.T. goals as it applies to weight reduction. The adjectives used for S.M.A.R.T. have different meanings for different variations depending on the circumstances and purposes. For weight reduction, S.M.A.R.T. is defined as:

S= specific
M= measurable
A= attainable
R= realistic or reasonable
T = trackable, timely (time-based) or tangible.

If you want to exercise you might say, "I'll exercise every day starting now." This is unrealistic. Very few, if any, people can exercise every day, seven days a week. A more realistic approach might be to say, "I'll exercise three times per week for 30 minutes." Rather than saying, "I'll eat vegetables more frequently," you might restate it as "I'll eat a minimum of one serving of veggies at lunch and one at dinner every day for the next two weeks." Clarity about reducing your weight and how you go about it is extremely important.

Are you starting to understand the importance of being clear on what you want to accomplish? The overall objective is to lose weight. But how you do it is the key. Setting time frames to modify or change your eating behavior is helpful. It gives direction and a plan to execute. Measuring your progress frequently is as important as establishing the goal. If you can quantify your results, you can objectively determine your success.

For example, the goal of eating healthier is not easily gauged. What does that mean? It means different things to different people. But, a target of eating 1,200 calories per day is quantifiable. You can get even more specific by breaking down the 1,200 calories into the amount of protein, healthy fats, carbohydrates, sugars, and fiber you'll get in the 1,200 calories.

Riding your bicycle more often is not calculable. What does that mean to you to ride your bicycle more often? If you haven't been on a bike in years and then ride it for a few days in the next month, does that satisfy your goal? Probably not. However, riding your bicycle for 45 minutes on Monday, Wednesday, and Friday is easy to assess.

Set an attainable goal for yourself. If you have doubts about achieving your goal, you're setting yourself up for failure. Many people declare they will work out every day. This might not be achievable if you know your work schedule won't permit it or your family obligations with the kids or grandkids will prevent you from working out every day. A more manageable expectation might be working out three days each week for 15 minutes. Be realistic when setting your weight-loss goal. Your goal should be sustainable and pragmatic given your resources and time. Focus on a result you can attain with some effort. If you have a bigger goal, break it into smaller more manageable phases. Attempting to achieve unreasonable aspirations will only set you up for failure.

Make sure there is a specific time frame to achieve your desired results. This provides a sense of urgency to accomplish your weight reduction target date. If you don't set a time frame to accomplish your weight-reduction goal, you'll never get there. As the Nike slogan said, "Yesterday you said tomorrow." We all know tomorrow never comes. It took me four months to shed 50 pounds. But I failed to do that during the previous eight years because I kept putting it off.

Make a list of reasons or benefits to accomplish your goal to reduce weight. This will help you keep engaged in your weight-loss process. For instance, the number one reason people reduce weight is for health reasons. Maybe you have high blood pressure, or maybe you are borderline diabetic.

Would you like to shed enough weight so that your doctor tells you there is no need to keep taking your prescription medication? How cool would that be?

In my situation, I needed to drop the weight to avoid having a heart attack, lower my cholesterol, and improve my overall health.

The number two reason people lose weight is to look better.

Do you want to lose weight because you have a special event to attend in the future? Maybe a class reunion, a wedding, or a vacation at a tropical resort and you want to look good in your swimsuit?

Do you find that being overweight is affecting your mobility? Do you think if you got rid of some extra weight, you'd feel better? Have more energy? Maybe your knees wouldn't hurt walking up a flight of stairs?

Determining a goal without knowing why or without having a reason to do it is a recipe for failure. Merely wanting to reduce weight is not enough. Most overweight individuals want to reduce weight. Acting and having goal-directed behavior is required to do so. Unfortunately, most people aren't successful in either starting these behavior modifications or maintaining them.

An effective behavioral modification technique, referred to as the "If this, then this" process", was originated by psychologist Peter Gollwitzer. The idea behind this concept is to have a plan for a specific situation that lends itself to being better able to handle the situation. The if this/ then this process helps you to deal with obstacles that might hinder you from accomplishing your goal. For example, let's imagine this hurdle pops-up. You're going to your friend's home and she is baking cookies. A specific, concrete and procedural approach might be to think, "When my friend asks me to indulge in eating a cookie with her, I will politely decline her invitation." Practice responding to any given situation you perceive as an obstacle before it occurs.

Another external obstacle might be that you're going to a fine Italian restaurant with friends. You can anticipate and expect the waiter to bring bread to the table. In applying the If this/then this process you'd anticipate your response. That being the situation, when the waiter brings bread to your table (if this) then you could ask to keep the bread at the opposite end of the table, turn your bread dish upside so as not to take a piece, drink more water, or simply decline any.

Often when my wife and I go out for dinner we instruct the waiter not to bring bread to the table. The reason for this is to be prepared before the situation arises. Find a phrase or tactic that works best for you in challenging situations.

Once you start acting to reach your goal, you'll find that you'll eventually attain it. Keeping a positive attitude is important no matter how small the weight reduction or what seems to be inconsequential or insignificant. Celebrate all wins no matter how small. We celebrate a lot of things – birthdays, anniversaries, and holidays – but when it comes to our accomplishments, we don't celebrate them all that often. It's important to celebrate your small victories because celebrating your wins makes you feel great and it reinforces the positive behavior you want to show up when you face a new challenge or obstacle.

Overlooking your successes can cause you to subconsciously take a negative view of your accomplishments. It's a universal law that when you focus on what you haven't accomplished instead of what you have, you are less likely to stay on task and complete your goals. What you focus on expands.

Celebrating your accomplishments can boost your confidence, help stave off lethargy, and motivate your continued success. Having the habit of celebrating successes, achievements, and wins, no matter how small or inconsequential they might seem, will help you to:

Learn and Adapt

You'll start to recognize what's working for you and why. This will help you to take something from it to inspire you or replicate in other actions and goals. Basically, you can accomplish more successes and achievements.

Ask yourself these four questions to debrief yourself:

- What happened? **Facts**
- How does that make you feel? **Feelings**
- What can you learn from this? **Findings**
- How will you use this going forward? (If you do not know, what would you tell someone who experienced the same situation?) **Future**

The Four F's: Facts, Feelings, Findings, Future

What emotions are you feeling?

1. Frustrated
2. Angry
3. Confused
4. Sad
5. Reluctant

Once you determine the emotion, ask yourself what you can do to alleviate your emotion in that situation. As an example, if you're feeling frustrated because you indulged in a pizza with friends, how can you alleviate your frustration? One way to do this is not to beat yourself up. No one is perfect. So, what happened? You ate some pizza.

How did it make you feel? Frustrated

What did you learn from this? Not to be frustrated or upset.

How will you use what you learned in the future? Have one slice of pizza instead of two. Or, take a few bites and leave the rest on the plate so it looks like you're eating it when you're not.

There are many different scenarios. Figure out what works best for you. It takes a lot of practice until it becomes automatic. Athletes spend hours and hours practicing.

Develop a Success Mindset

A large part of weight-reduction success is about your state of mind. That's why it's important to have a success mindset because when you position yourself as a winner, you open the door for more success to come your way. Bill Carmody, Founder, and CEO of Trepoint said, "Success begets success, so it's only natural to build upon existing momentum, especially during events of celebration. Perception becomes reality."

When you've achieved a small weight loss or a smaller dress size or tightened your belt another notch, instead of immediately moving on to the next thing of your long list of things to do, take a moment, spend some time to reflect on what you've achieved, and celebrate it. A small celebration can be making a fist with your right hand, bringing your elbow down towards your hip while saying "Yes!"

Have you have seen this done by others?

Celebrating Accomplishments Builds Your Confidence

Would you like to be even more confident? Celebrating your small victories and telling yourself that you can reduce weight, feel better, and have more energy will do wonders for your confidence. Instead of downplaying your achievement, attributing it to luck or giving others credit, acknowledge them. It's important to do this because it acts as a reminder of your success and that you can achieve even more.

Celebrating Small Wins Will Increase Your Motivation

If you don't celebrate your small wins and achievements, it's easy to lose motivation and can cause you to give up, quit. Celebrating helps you stay motivated because it acts as a reward. And, you should reward yourself, but not with an ice cream sundae or other foods. Instead, purchase a new dress, pair of shoes, or another tangible item other than food. It can be something as simple as a pen or knick-knack. Being positive and celebrating has a cumulative effect of sustaining your momentum and keeping you motivated instead of discouraged.

Celebrating Releases Happiness

Have you ever noticed you feel good when you celebrate? That's because when you celebrate dopamine, is released into your brain. Achieving small goals and celebrating them releases more dopamine which causes us to feel happy. The more you feel this positive emotion, the more you want to feel this way. Dr. B.J. Fogg, an experimental psychologist at Stanford, explained it this way when he said, "Emotions create habits ... when you complete your tiny habit, reward yourself with an 'Awesome!' or 'Good for me!' to affirm to yourself this is a behavior you're proud of."

Inspire Others by Celebrating Your Success

You can inspire others by celebrating your achievements. Seeing you accomplish your goals might motivate others. So, whether you go to the movies or buy yourself something you've been wanting or just take some time to do things that you enjoy, make sure you find a way to celebrate.

Let's review the three primary reasons why celebrating your wins is so critically important to your weight-reduction success.

#1: The Act of Celebrating Changes Your Physiology and Strengthens Your Psychology

When you celebrate, endorphins, specifically, dopamine, are released inside your body and you feel incredible. When you accomplish something and don't take the time to celebrate, you are robbing yourself of an important feeling that reinforces your success. So much of what we do in your weight-loss journey and lifestyle transformation is driven (or limited) by our psychology. Celebrating your wins not only feels great physically, but it reinforces the behavior you want to show up when you face a new challenge or opportunity.

Conversely, if you fail to celebrate your many accomplishments, you are training your brain that what you are doing isn't all that exciting and important. If every day feels mundane (even when you are crushing it), you will stop giving 110 percent of yourself and that will lead to lackluster results. Simply put, the lack of celebration will lead to a feeling of emptiness that will result in less focus and decreased performance over time.

#2: Celebrating with Colleagues and Friends Tightens Your Network

By no means must you throw a party to celebrate. There are many psychological and physiological benefits in simply acknowledging your wins (either in a journal or with a close friend or family member). But there are added benefits when you expand your circle to include your colleagues or others on their weight-reduction journey.

Your own celebration is contagious and those around you will want to share in your success. As your weight-loss accomplishments are celebrated, new ideas for healthy meals and snacks are shared. In a peak state, you feel you can accomplish anything. When surrounded by others who are also in a peak state, it's natural to look for ways to collaborate and strengthen your network of weight-loss achievers.

#3: Your Celebrations Position You Correctly as A Winner and Attracts More Success

Success begets more success, so it's only natural to build upon existing momentum; especially during events of celebration. As you look to shed your unwanted extra weight, celebratory events not only reinforce the positive aspects of what you are doing, but positions yourself as a person with whom others would like to associate. Perception becomes reality. As you celebrate your wins, others look for ways to participate in what you have successfully done. The right partnerships are formed. This means that you attract others who successfully reduced weight and enjoy a more active lifestyle. There is a high probability you will make new connections and new friends. There is also a possibility that former friends who have not enjoyed your transformation accomplishment might be jealous and envious.

Chapter 9

Applying the Wisdom of Vince Lombardi to Reducing Weight

Life's battles don't always go to the stronger or faster man. But sooner or later, the man who wins is the man who thinks he can.

Vince Lombardi

In this chapter, you will learn how the wisdom of legendary NFL Green Bay Packer's coach Vince Lombardi can be applied to reduce weight.

Vince Lombardi was an American football player, coach, and executive in the National Football League (NFL). He is best known as the head coach of the Green Bay Packers during the 1960s, where he led the team to three straight and five total NFL Championships in seven years in addition to winning the first two Super Bowls at the conclusion of the 1966 and 1967 NFL seasons. Following his sudden death from cancer in 1970, the NFL Super Bowl trophy was named to honor him. Lombardi was enshrined in the Pro Football Hall of Fame in 1971, the year after his death. Lombardi is considered by most to be the greatest coach in football history. He is so inspirational that many of his quotes are used by many companies in various businesses as well as life coaches.

Lombardi said, "Once a man has made a commitment to a way of life, he puts the greatest strength in the world behind him. It's something we call heart power. Once a man has made a commitment, nothing will stop him short of success."

This Lombardi quote has nothing to do with football and everything to do with commitment. With respect to losing weight, once you have made a commitment to reducing weight in a healthy and sustainable manner, you'll put forth your greatest strength in the world and nothing will stop you short of success. Your commitment to anything in life, especially as it applies to weight loss, will determine your success. Lombardi focused a lot on commitment. He said, "There is only one way to succeed in anything and that is to give it everything."

If you want to succeed in anything, including losing weight, make a commitment to do it and you will succeed. If you're not willing to reduce weight, no one can help you. If you are determined to shed those extra unwanted and unhealthy pounds, no one can stop you.

Napoleon Hill, author of *Think and Grow Rich*, referred to this as a burning desire. You must have a burning desire or a compelling reason to reduce weight. A half-hearted effort will never produce positive results. What has it cost you by not acting and implementing small adjustments to your daily eating routines to improve your eating habits and shed your unwanted pounds?

Do your knees hurt because of your excess weight?

Are you constantly tired?

Do you make excuses not to play with your kids or grandkids?

Once you steadfastly commit to reducing weight and are resolute in your efforts to do so, the universe will assist you, guide you, support you, and even create miracles for you.

Lombardi said, "The quality of a person's life is in direct proportion to their commitment to excellence, regardless of their chosen field of endeavor."

Applying Lombardi's philosophy to reducing weight, might be re-phrased as, "The quality of a person's health is in direct proportion to their commitment to maintaining a healthy weight."

Lombardi also said, "Winning is not a sometime thing; it's an all the time thing. You don't win occasionally, you don't do things right once in a while, you do them right all of the time. Winning is a habit. Unfortunately, so is losing." Reducing weight is a lifestyle change and a lifetime endeavor. It's not like getting a vaccine where you get a shot and you're done for the rest of your life. Rephrasing this quote, you can say, "Maintaining a healthy weight is not a sometime thing; it's an all the time thing. You don't lose weight in a healthy way occasionally. You reduce weight in a healthy manner and keep it off. Reducing weight is based on habits. Unfortunately, so is gaining weight."

Zig Ziglar said, "People often say that motivation doesn't last. Well, neither does bathing - that's why we recommend it daily." Applying the analogy of taking a bath or shower to weight reduction, you can't take a bath or shower once and be done with it. You need to do it daily. To reduce weight and keep it off you need to eat healthy and drink pure water each day.

You learned about habits and making small changes and improvements to your daily eating routines and habits in a previous chapter. Lombardi said, "The only place success comes before work is in the dictionary." Achieving and maintaining a healthy weight is work. If anyone tells you differently, they're either naturally blessed with an awesome body or they're lying.

You'll be challenged every day by food companies, restaurants, fast food chains, and social gatherings with friends and families. Images of people enjoying food and alcoholic beverages and sodas are everywhere – TV ads, magazines, newspapers, online, billboards. Food and drink are constantly pushed in front of you.

Lombardi said, "Don't succumb to excuses. Go back to the job of making the corrections and forming the habits that will make your goal possible." Do you believe forming good habits is necessary to achieving a healthy weight that you can maintain? According to Lombardi, stop making excuses. If you have a setback, correct your mistake and keep moving forward to improve your eating habits each day. We all justify and have explanations or reasons for not reducing weight or maintaining it. You'll either have excuses or you'll have results. It's your choice.

Another of my favorite quotes from Lombardi is, "Life's battles don't always go to the stronger or faster man. But sooner or later, the man who wins is the man who thinks he can." Applying these words to reducing weight, "The weight-loss battles don't always go to the person with the most willpower or discipline. But sooner or later, the people who can lose weight and keep it off are the people who think they can."

It's been said that practice makes perfect. Wrong! Practice only makes a habit. Hall of Fame Quarterback Joe Montana told the story that when he played for the San Francisco 49ers, they didn't practice a play until they got it right, they practiced it until they didn't get it wrong.

It was Vince Lombardi who said, "Practice does not make perfect. Only perfect practice makes perfect."

Let's be honest. No one is perfect. But we can all strive to get better. Professional athletes will always say they can get better. Vince Lombardi expressed it best when he said, "Perfection is not attainable, but if we chase perfection, we can catch excellence."

Would you like to achieve and maintain excellent health? If so, what are you doing about it?

Michael Jordan, arguably the best, or at least one of the best basketball players to play the game, always strived to be better. It was that mentality that drove him to be one of the best, if not the best. Jordan knew what he accomplished wasn't where he stopped. There was always room to improve. Likewise, with our eating habits, there is always room to improve. It doesn't mean we need to do things perfectly. It just means that small improvements to our daily eating routines done consistently over a long time will give us noticeable and sustainable results.

Here is an acronym you can use: STIED. It stands for Strive to Improve Each (or every) Day.

Lombardi said, "Success is like anything worthwhile. It has a price. You must pay the price to win and you have to pay the price to get to the point where success is possible. Most important, you must pay the price to stay there." You can never own your weight-loss success. You can only rent it. And the rent is due every day in the form of the food and beverage choices we choose to eat and drink.

During the 2017 NBA playoffs, a commentator for game four between the Cleveland Cavaliers and the Toronto Raptors mentioned Lebron James, also arguably the best basketball player. According to the commentator, James arrived at the stadium before any other player and went through a complete workout in preparation for the game. James habitually stayed an extra 45 minutes to an hour after practice and was the last player to leave the court. James stated, "You have to put in the work if you expect to improve your game." Similarly, if you want to reduce weight and keep it off, and achieve better health, you need to put forth the effort to make it happen.

I'll repeat what I said earlier, with respect to weight: you can never own your weight-loss success. You can only rent it. And the rent is due every day in the form of the food and beverages we choose to eat and drink. It comes down to the choices you make.

Lombardi said, "The measure of who we are is what we do with what we have." The measure of who you are as it pertains to your weight can be measured by what you choose to do to properly nourish your body. Is it worth it to you to put forth the time and effort to purchase the ingredients for a healthy meal and to take the time to prepare it? Or will you be like the majority who'd just go through the drive-thru or pick up a bucket of fried chicken?

How often do you choose convenience over health? When it comes to results, Lombardi said, "Some of us will do our jobs well, some will not. But we will be judged by only one thing – the result." Maybe you will commit to modifying and improving your eating behaviors and habits. Maybe you won't. Maybe you will make better food and beverage choices, maybe you won't. You will, however, be judged by your weight-reduction results. Hopefully you will achieve a healthy weight and maintain it. Maybe you won't. We shall see if you will succeed or not. Lombardi taught, "Winning is a habit. Watch your thoughts, they become your beliefs. Watch your beliefs, they become your words. Watch your words, they become your actions. Watch your actions, they become your habits. Watch your habits, they become your character."

One of the world's most renowned architects, Frank Lloyd Wright, designed over 1,000 structures and finished more than 500 of them. Towards the end of his career, he was asked which was his favorite of all his beautiful creations. Without hesitating, he replied, "My next one."

Despite accomplishing so much, Wright recognized that he wasn't done and there was more to achieve. He comprehended the fact that even though he had tremendous success, there was something greater for him to do. This mindset and type of perspective, much like Lombardi, pushed him throughout his entire career.

Too often, instead of striving to be our best, we settle for mediocrity. Are you content to be average? Do you want to be your best? To be in the best health possible? No matter where you're starting with respect to your weight, you've only just begun to accomplish great things and achieve lifelong optimal health. Don't ever stop striving to be your best. You might surprise yourself as you move forward to your "next one."

Achieving better health is a mindset. Vince Lombardi said, "If you'll not settle for anything less than your best, you will be amazed at what you can accomplish in your lives." He also said, "Winning means you're willing to go longer, work harder, and give more than anyone else." Winning your weight issue means you're willing to forgo certain foods and beverages that others are enjoying and eat healthier foods that others might ignore. Again, you are not sacrificing or depriving yourself of anything. You are making a conscientious decision to eat healthier.

Imagine viewing food as fuel for your body instead of for comfort. Is there a legitimate reason you don't want to put the best fuel in your body for optimal performance? You can accomplish this simply by avoiding processed foods, eating more whole or holistic foods, and drinking more pure water. There are powers inside each of us that, if we tap into them and use them, we can make our healthy weight journey more successful than we can ever have imagined or dreamed we could accomplish. You can achieve and maintain a healthy weight. I'm proof, along with thousands and thousands of others, that transformation is possible.

Vince Lombardi spoke about success and what is required. He said, "The price of success is hard work, dedication to the job at hand, and the determination that whether we win or lose, we have applied the best of ourselves to the task at hand." Are you applying the best of yourself to succeed at reducing weight? Be honest with yourself.

Unfortunately, a consequence of not getting rid of your unhealthy pounds, not accomplishing the task at hand, could be premature death. Keep in mind more people are dying from health issues related to being overweight than from smoking. And, more than 71 percent of the U.S. adult population is overweight, of which 40 percent is clinically obese.

Les Brown said, "The graveyard is the richest place on earth because it is here that you will find all the hopes and dreams that were never fulfilled, the books that were never written. The songs that were never sung, the inventions that were never shared, the cures that were never discovered, all because someone was too afraid to take the first step, keep with the problem, or determined to carry out their dream." Imagine your hopes and dreams were cut short because you failed to take care of yourself by simply reducing weight and making better food choices. It would be very sad if you had a heart attack or stroke, or a chronic illness that prevented you from accomplishing your potential. All of which could have been avoided by making a lifestyle change.

If the wisdom of Vince Lombardi and several others mentioned during this lesson don't motivate you to act to shed your unwanted and unhealthy pounds, nothing will. Will it take you being told you have a 95 percent chance for a fatal heart attack to wake up, like I did, and do something?

Here are several questions for you to contemplate:
- What is your greatest challenge to reducing your weight?
- If you've started, what's working?
- What's not working?
- What about reducing is important to you?
- What are you wanting to accomplish by reducing weight?
- What is your biggest obstacle to moving forward?

Imagine what you could do if you weighed less and felt better. Imagine having more energy and more confidence because you feel and look better.

Chapter 10

Learning from Mistakes –
Why Failure is Important

*What makes us happy is seeing the
evidence of progress.*

In this chapter, we will delve into some deep thoughts and ideas. It usually takes more than one reading to digest all the concepts, so you may want to revisit this chapter.

Have you made mistakes? Of course, you have. We all have. But, did you learn from your mistakes? That's the question.

In this chapter you'll learn why making mistakes is important in weight-reduction. Can we agree that we all learn by trial and error? You need to figure out what will work for you and what won't when it comes to achieving a healthy weight.

Do you feel it's better to learn from the mistakes of others rather than your own mistakes? You might be surprised to learn that yes; it actually is better to learn from the mistakes of others. We'll get into the reason in a moment.

In the meantime, it's important to understand that the one mechanism humans have developed to avoid making the same mistake over and over is the spoken word, the written word; otherwise known as language. The word is a shortcut to passing along information from one generation to the next, because words convey concepts.

Here's an example. Translators in Europe are very fast. They can translate almost simultaneously as something is being said. Translators in China are a little slower. Translators in Vietnam, however, are very slow.

Why are translators in Vietnam slow compared to those in China and Europe? The reason is that Vietnam has fewer words to convey or explain concepts in their language. Until recently,

Vietnam was a rural country of mostly agriculture and little technology. So it takes longer to explain an idea.

R. Buckminster (Bucky) Fuller wrote an article touching on language and words for *Intuition* magazine, titled "Mistake Mystique." Bucky Fuller was a 20th-century inventor and visionary who published more than 30 books. Fuller did not limit himself to one field but worked as a "comprehensive anticipatory design scientist" to solve global problems. Fuller's ideas and work continue to influence new generations of designers, architects, scientists, and artists.

One notion gleaned from the *Mistake Mystique* article is that in addition to the basic needs of food, water, shelter, and nurturing, we need to be curious to learn. He said being curious to learn is a basic human need. Fuller surmised that to survive as a species, it's necessary to multiply and to develop words as a short cut to explain concepts to help future generations to avoid the same mistakes.

Let me provide an example to illustrate this point. Imagine you travel back in time to ancient Rome. How would you communicate the concept of an automobile, an airplane, or a rocket ship? Today, you can do this using one word. You can understand what is being communicated to you when you hear the word automobile, airplane, or rocket ship. We may have different visualizations of what is being conveyed, but the concept is understood. But, back in ancient Rome, you'd need more words to convey the concepts of these modern-day terms. This is the reason it takes longer for translators in Vietnam to translate what is being said. They need to explain the concept.

Life is a journey of making mistakes. And that's a good thing, so long as we learn from them. The word "mistake" unfairly means something bad or negative. This is a misconception. How you perceive the word "Mistake" is the meaning you've been taught or the connotation that you've given it. But, there's a difference between a *fact* and an *opinion* that determines your perception.

A *fact* is a thing that is known or proven to be true. An *opinion* is a belief or judgment that falls short of absolute conviction, certainty, or positive knowledge; a belief, judgment, or way of thinking about something; what someone thinks about a thing that has not been proven true and remains open to dispute. And, perception is a belief or opinion, often held by many people and based on how things seem, the way that you think about it, or the impression you have of it.

The definition of "mistake" is an action or judgment that is misguided or wrong. Just because it is incorrect, does not make it bad. That it is bad might be your perception, but it is open to be disputed.

In the movie *National Treasure*, Nicholas Cage playing Benjamin Gates said, "You know, Thomas Edison tried and failed nearly 2,000 times to develop the carbonized cotton filament for the incandescent lightbulb. And when asked about it he said, 'I didn't fail. I found 2,000 ways how not to make a light bulb,' but he only needed to find one way to make it work."

Edison didn't look at the mistakes of finding the correct way to make the carbonized cotton filament as bad or negative. He saw them as learning opportunities. What is wrong with making a mistake if that is how we learn? At the beginning of this chapter, I asked if we could all agree that we learn from mistakes, ours and others'. Being wrong about something does not necessarily translate into it being bad or negative. It's important to view a miscalculation, misunderstanding, oversight, or something misconstrued as a positive, a learning opportunity to figure out the one way or several ways to get it right.

This applies to weight loss. There are many ways to lose weight. You only need to figure out the one way for you to reduce weight in a healthy manner that you can sustain.

Hollywood gives a great explanation for why "miss-takes" are valuable. In filming a movie or TV series, Hollywood uses a clapperboard to mark the beginning of a segment for editing purposes. A clapperboard makes a loud sound. It's used in filmmaking and video production to help synchronize the picture with the sound or audio. It also designates the various scenes as they are being recorded.

In cinematography, a "take" refers to each filmed version of a particular scene or "shot." "Takes" are generally numbered starting with "take one" and are numbered in successive order with the director calling for "take two" or "take fifteen" until the filming is completed. A miss-take (missed take) or outtake is a scene not used in the edited version of a film or videotape. In other words, a mistake. Actors and directors do many takes to get the scene right. They're learning to get the scene correct from mistakes. They do many takes before getting it right. So why should a mistake be viewed or construed as "bad" or a negative if it's a learning tool used in Hollywood?

Unlike Hollywood, teachers can stunt a child's learning development by punishing them for a mistake. If you make an error answering a question on a test you're marked down. Why won't teachers allow a student to learn from the mistake, re-take the exam or quiz and get credit for realizing what they did wrong? Haven't we agreed that learning comes from making mistakes and correcting ourselves?

How does it help a child learn to make them feel "bad" if they do poorly on a test or quiz? It doesn't. The only thing a child learns is that it's "bad" to make a mistake. In business when two or more companies or individuals get together to solve a problem, it's called collaboration. Yet, if students get together to solve a problem, it's called cheating.

Life is a journey of making mistakes. We learn by trial and error. Your best teacher is your last mistake. This might be why so many of us have a negative connotation or perception of the word "mistake." Are you willing to admit your mistakes when it comes to reducing weight, so you can learn and achieve your goal or objective more quickly?

If words have impact and words are developed to communicate concepts, then it's important to understand the etymology of some words. Etymology is the study of the origin of words and the way in which their meanings have changed throughout history.

As an example, let's look at the etymology of the word "sin." In a religious context, "sin" is an act of transgression against divine or natural law. Sin can also be viewed as any thought or action that endangers the ideal relationship between an individual and God; or as any diversion from the perceived ideal order for human living.

Upon further examination, the word "sin" derives from "Old English "syn", which meant to go astray. The word "sin" means to miss the mark. The English Biblical terms translated as "sin" or "syn" from the Biblical Greek and Jewish terms sometimes originate from words in the latter languages denoting the act or state of missing the mark. The original sense of New Testament Greek "sin" is failure, being in error, missing the mark, especially in spear throwing.

In Hebrew, the word "sin" originated in archery and literally refers to missing the "gold" at the center of a target, but hitting the target, i.e. error. "To sin" has been defined from a Greek concordance as "to miss the mark."

Bucky Fuller said, "Mistakes are sins only when not admitted." Once you admit the mistake you can receive the lesson to be learned from the universe.

We all make mistakes every day, but you still might not view them as learning opportunities. In this chapter you'll be taught several powerful lessons you can acquire from making a mistake.

1. **A mistake teaches you to clarify what you really want and how you want to live**. The word mistake gets its meaning from you. You give it meaning. The word mistake can be perceived differently by each person. How many of you compare mistake with success?

Noticing and admitting your mistakes along your weight-reduction journey helps you stay in touch with your commitment – what you want to accomplish, and what you need to do shed those unwanted pounds.

A mistake is like a flashing sign that says, "improve or change this." The urgency is to focus on the obstacles or challenges preventing you from making different choices when deciding what to eat or which beverage to drink. Re-examining why we made a choice to indulge can help get you back on track, provide clarity and help stay positive to improve next time the situation occurs.

2. **A mistake teaches you to be honest with yourself.** It's natural to want to hide our mistake if we eat what we know we shouldn't like a slice of pizza or several pieces of bread served at the

restaurant because we get embarrassed by a lack of discipline. But being honest with yourself is an opportunity to improve the next time. It's like holding up a mirror to yourself and really seeing. What you do in private your wear in public. You're not fooling anyone other than yourself. So, ask yourself what happened? (I ate some bread). How did it make you feel? (I felt guilty). What can we learn from this experience? (Be honest with the decision and not hide it). How can you use what you learned in the future? Avoid bread at the restaurant by asking the server to not bring any or keep it at the other end of the table, or drink water instead of munching on the bread. Being honest with yourself will help you concentrate on letting go of the embarrassment to learn. It's not what you do when people are watching, it's what you do in private when no one is watching – except yourself.

3. **A mistake will teach you to accept your fallibility**. Sometimes even your best efforts just don't work out. We all have good intentions to lose weight. You might have tried a diet and failed and tried another and failed again. When this happens, admit you're stuck. Ask for support. Ask someone to keep you accountable. When you admit you're stuck and are unable to do it alone, it sends a signal and opens the door for help to show. Solutions, resources, even a person might appear in your life to help you resolve the issue of being overweight.

4. **A mistake can teach you, through analysis and feedback, what's working and what's not working**. It's your reality check. By making a mistake, you'll learn what doesn't work on the path to reducing weight and learn or find out what will work for you.

The feedback you get from your mistake can be the most specific and meaningful information you'll receive. Often, you can trace a mistake to behaviors or beliefs that can be changed and improved.

Maybe you'll have that "ah-ha" moment by filtering your mistake through a series of questions: "How can I use this experience to improve?", "What will I do differently next time?", "How will I be different in the future?" Questions like these lead to an inquiry that invites solutions.

5. **A mistake can teach you to be accountable**. Our instinctive reaction when we make a mistake is to shift blame rather than accept responsibility and learn from it. It's more empowering for you to accept your role in making a mistake, learn from it and move on. Shifting the blame on others won't help you. Remember, it's about understanding what you can do differently next time. Delving into the mistake instead of ignoring it or shifting blame reminds you that you have choices and your actions have a huge influence on your weight-loss success. Anything is possible. You have options. I respect your choices. Keep in mind, Emerson said, "Your actions speak so loud I cannot hear what you are saying."

6. **A mistake says a lot about your integrity**. A mistake will often happen because you break your promise, overcommit, or agree to avoid conflict. How many of you promised you'd lose weight? How many of you kept your promise? How many of you committed to exercising more or eating more fruits and vegetables? How many of you said you'd eat less processed food? These are examples of breaking a promise or over committing.

By now, hopefully, you'll have started to implement the information you were given in the previous lessons.

Big mistakes generally start as small errors. Gaining weight starts by making choices to eat differently. It's more convenient to pick up food at a drive-thru than prepare a meal at home. We're tired, hungry, and we become complacent. Over time, these tiny choices accumulate and show on our waistline or with us ending up with a medical ailment.

When we stay in our integrity to improve our eating habits, we pay attention to the choices we make each day. The nearer we live to the source of health the more health we shall receive. A mistake can be a signal that our words are out of alignment with our actions. If this happens, you can re-examine your intentions, reconsider your commitment, and adjust your actions.

Your history does not predict your future. Anything is possible. You have options. I respect your choices. When confronted with making a mistake while attempting to reduce weight do you pull back, retreat? Instead, rise to the challenge, figure out a way to overcome the obstacle preventing your weight loss and move forward.

Your mistake can inspire others. After all, were you inspired by my weight-reduction story of shedding 50 pounds in four months? Are you inspired by others who are successfully dropping weight? Does that inspire you to commit to doing the same?

Let's examine how failure can help you with your weight-loss journey. We've all experienced failure at some point in our lives. J.K. Rowling said, "It is impossible to live without failing at something unless you live so cautiously that you might as well not have lived at all, in which case you have failed by default."

Failure is defined as a lack of success; the fact of not doing something that you must do or are expected to do. According to the English Oxford Dictionary, failure is a lack of success, the neglect or omission of expected or required action, the action or state of not functioning. So why is failure necessary to be successful? Because failure is like a mistake. It is through your failures that you can learn your greatest lessons in life.

Do you think about failure in a negative light?

Yes, failure is painful. Yes, it causes emotional turmoil and upset. Yes, it inflicts agonizing pangs of shame, grief, and distress. But those who have bounced back from true failure, understand that failure is necessary for success. If you're not tested by adversity, you might not realize your full potential. If you're not tested by adversity to reduce weight and shed your unwanted pounds, you might be content to remain overweight.

Being overweight is a failure. It is the failure of not drinking enough pure water and eating healthier. Yet, your failure can help you find your determination to successfully lose weight and keep it off.

Here's an example. When a baby is learning to walk, it will fall down often. This is a failure. But every mother knows that their baby will walk one day. The baby will fall down many times, but it will walk. Why is a mother so confident that her child will walk? Because, as we all know, falling down and failing while learning to walk is just a part of life. It's normal to learn from our failure. It's like riding a bicycle. Were you able to hop on a bike and ride it the first time? Unless it had training wheels, probably not.

What we don't realize is some people, like me, had to go through the experience of gaining and losing weight, to get to where they are in life as it relates to weight. Let me explain. Like many of you, I wasn't always overweight. I was fit and trim. But, as with many of you, life happened. Before I realized it, I had gained a lot of weight. I had to experience the failure of gaining weight to experience the success of reducing weight.

If I hadn't gained the weight, I could not relate to you what it feels like to be overweight. I couldn't relate to you how it feels to be embarrassed by your weight. Or, how it feels to fail to lose weight after turning from one diet to another. To succeed, I had to fail. Now, I'm driven by my fear of failure to maintain a healthy weight. After all, how would it look for a weight-reduction specialist to be overweight?

Here's the rub. Society tends to celebrate the success rather than highlighting the heroic journeys achieving success, the setbacks, upsets, and failures it took. It's not glamorous to talk about getting fired from a job only to succeed in starting a business. It's not appealing for me to look at photos of myself when I was overweight. Rachel Gillet wrote, "What may initially feel like failure may just be the launching pad needed for success."

J.K. Rowling, when she was a secretary for the London office of Amnesty International, spent too much time at work writing about a teenage wizard named Harry Potter. Rowling secretly wrote her stories on her work computer and daydreamed about being a writer. Her employer got fed up and terminated her employment. Her severance check helped support her over the next few years.

The original Harry Potter manuscript was rejected by 12 publishing houses before Bloomsbury picked it up. Michael Jordan expressed failure another way: "I've missed more than 9,000 shots in my career. I've lost almost 300 games. 26 times, I've been trusted to take the game winning shot and missed. I've failed over and over and over again in my life. And that's why I succeed." So, are you ready to learn from your weight-loss failures, otherwise known as diets, to modify your lifestyle and improve your eating habits?

Think of failure as a stepping stone. You'll learn several powerful life lessons that failure helps to instill in us and teach. If you've failed to lose weight and keep it off, and you're going through a rough time right now, keep these important lessons in mind.

An Important Lesson Gained From Failure is Experience

What happens when you fail? You gain first-hand experience. Your journey through life is based on your experiences. Failure brings you knowledge that can be used for future situations.

Failure in Life Builds Resilience

The more you fail, the more resilient you become. For you to achieve weight-loss success, you must know how to be resilient. Because if you think you're going to succeed reducing weight the first attempt you make, you're mistaken. Resilience is being persistent. You must be persistent to reduce weight, to keep making improved food choices. To keep moving forward when you have an off moment or day.

Failure creates value

In thinking about your past failures, think about how much value you bring with you to the table. You're able to share your knowledge gained from your past failures and that makes you valuable.

Once you comprehend the value of failure and how it's meant to serve you rather than hinder you, your mind and heart are open to experience failure. Ultimately, you'll have to decide what is a failure. What you might consider a failure, say, losing 20 pounds, another might see that as a success. But it doesn't matter how others view your weight-reduction journey. What matters is how you view it and what you consider success.

When you reach a plateau and haven't lost as much weight as you set as a goal, there will be people telling you, "I told you so," and "I knew you wouldn't do it." Maybe one of those voices in your own head. Ignore these people. Be resilient. Be persistent. Keep making those small adjustments consistently to your daily eating routine and after a long time, a few months, you'll see noticeable results. Those who said you couldn't or wouldn't do it will be envious of your results.

It's OK to fail. But it's not OK to give up. Success will taste so much sweeter when you reach your healthy weight. You'll look and feel amazing in that new outfit. You'll have more energy and be more confident.

Failure might take you on a path you might not want to travel on. But, the truth of the situation is that path will help shape you into a better person, a healthier person. Unfortunately, there is no path forward in life without experiencing failure. It's what you do with experiencing failure and applying the lessons learned that will determine your ultimate success.

Let's review how to debrief after failure. First, determine what happened. *The facts.* Next, how did this make you feel? *Your feelings.* Then, what did you learn from this failure? *The findings.* And, how can you apply what you learned from the failure to future situations or events? *The future.*

Your being overweight is a failure to eat healthy. Your being overweight and learning to eat healthier can be a great platform for personal development that is unmatched.

Without my being overweight and having to shed my unwanted and unhealthy pounds, I'd never have met the people I've met, been able to help so many other individuals reduce weight and learn to spot the weight-loss rhetoric being spewed by people wanting to take advantage of others for a profit. If you firmly believe in your weight-reduction goals, you can use the lessons learned from failure to push past your old limitations. Thomas Edison said, "If we did all the things, we are capable of, we would astound ourselves."

Chapter 11

Common Obstacles and Challenges to Reduce Weight

Warning, Warning, Danger, Will Robinson!
The Robot, *Lost in Space*

It's your decision what you put into your mouth.

It doesn't matter if you'd like to shed 10 pounds, 50 pounds, or over 100 pounds, it can feel like a million weight-loss obstacles standing in your way. Reducing weight in a healthy and sustainable manner in never easy. There are many mental, psychological, emotional, logistical, and lifestyle factors to conquer to achieve your weight-loss goal.

In this chapter, you will learn some of the most common challenges and obstacles that get in the way and how to overcome them.

One of the most common challenges you'll face is not having time to cook. No one denies it's easier to go get food at the fast food drive-thru or pick-up a bucket of fried chicken than to make something from scratch. But cooking healthy food doesn't necessarily require a lot of time.

Many tasty options, like a main course salad, don't require any cooking time. The key is to plan before your stomach starts rumbling. Tammy Lakatos, a certified dietician, personal trainer, and co-author of *The Nutrition Twins' Veggie Cure*, suggests taking time on the weekend to plan out meals for the next week. Be certain to chop up veggies and protein and keep them in the fridge. Use portion control containers as an easy way to make sure your food portions are proper.

After a long day at work, it's much faster to look in the fridge and pull out a container of the chopped veggies and protein to add to some mixed greens for a quick, healthy, and easy main course salad.

It'll probably take less time to prepare the salad than to stop for a takeout order.

A second obstacle or challenge is believing you'll be hungry all the time. You don't need to eat small amounts of food to reduce weight. The best way to feel full and reduce weight is to drink two 8-ounce glasses of water about 10 minutes before each meal. If you're unable to drink two full glasses, drink at least one 8-ounce glass without ice.

Another way to eat less and feel full is to fill up on whole grains, raw vegetables, fruits, and lean protein. Eat more vegetables than fruit. How much? You should eat three times more vegetables than fruit. Many people incorrectly believe that fruits and vegetables are the same and will consume ten fruits to one vegetable. They're not the same.

As an example, I have a few clients who will tell me they're having trouble losing weight and that they are doing everything correctly. But, when asked what they're eating, it turns out they are eating more fruits, sometimes a lot of fruit, then vegetables. After all, fruits are sweeter and contain more natural sugar than vegetables.

Fruits contain more natural sugar than vegetables. Berries, such as blueberries, blackberries, raspberries, and strawberries, are the exception. When it comes to berries, you can eat as much as you want. The reason being that berries have low calorie and high glycemic levels and they will fill you up. You'd have to eat an entire pint of blueberries to equal one regular-sized Hershey bar.

When you hear the words, "raw food diet," do you think of eating carrots and celery sticks all day long and being hungry all the time? That's a misconception of what it means to eat a "raw food diet." You'd be amazed at how creative you can be on a raw food diet. As an example, raw nuts such as walnuts, almonds, pecans, and cashews are a great source of protein. Avocados are loaded with fiber and a great source of potassium. Apples are delicious and make a great snack. Raw cheese is amazing.

Because your meal-prep time is limited, many of you like to microwave your food. You should NEVER use a microwave to cook or reheat your food.

With more than 90 percent of American households having microwaves, how many of you are wondering why I'd suggest never using a microwave? After all, microwaves are everywhere; in dorms, offices, break rooms, fast food places, restaurants, and every workplace. They're quick and easy, and the convenience they offer is undeniable. Plus, they don't take up much space. Because of this, you may be convinced that microwaved food poses no danger to you. That's what the microwave industry wants you to believe.

Do you believe because the government approves the use of microwaves that it must be safe? Extensive research for negative articles or information on the internet revealed that there are few to be found. So, it must be safe right? You're wrong.

In searching the internet for information about microwave food being harmful to consume, you'll find many articles that state otherwise. In other words, all the articles I reviewed stated that eating microwaved food was perfectly safe.

So, what gives?

According to Dr. Edward C. Kondrot, M.D., best-selling author of the *10 Essentials to Save Your Sight,* "The real dangers of microwave cooking have been systematically suppressed."

Dr. Kondrot is a world-leading homeopathic Ophthalmologist who devotes his practice to traditional and alternative therapies for the treatment of eye disease.

Why are microwave ovens a danger to your health? Because they alter the food's cellular makeup. In doing so, it alters your blood chemistry. The more often you consume food that has been microwaved, the more significant and permanent the damage becomes. Microwaves are part of the electromagnetic spectrum of energy that includes light and radio waves. Microwaves travel at the speed of light. The speed of light is about 186,282 miles per second. Micro wavelengths interact with molecules in the food being heated up. This interaction creates new, unnatural radiolytic compounds. These radiolytic compounds are not found in nature. These new foreign man-made compounds have been shown to cause damage to the blood, the digestive system, and other immune systems.

Extensive research to prove the dangers of eating microwaved food have been done in other countries such as Russia, Germany, and Switzerland. Their conclusions of the clinical studies found microwaved food can cause brain damage. The human body cannot metabolize, or breakdown, unknown byproducts found in microwaved food, and male and female hormone production is shut down or altered.

The dangerous effects of consuming microwaved food are comparable to smoking cigarettes. How long were cigarettes considered safe, glamorous, even fashionable, before the Surgeon General in 1965 stated it was a health hazard. Warnings were required on all cigarette packaging starting in 1970. The cumulative negative health side effects took years for a person to realize cigarette smoking is unhealthy. Likewise, you won't realize the dangerous health side effects of consuming microwaved food until after many, many years of eating it.

If you'd like to do more reading on your own, you can find some articles about the dangers of microwaved food at www.globalhealingcenter.com.

OK, let's get back to the question posed earlier, that being: Do you believe nutritious food is too expensive? You're probably wrong. Fast food combo meals cost between $6 to $8. It's cheaper to make a healthy meal at home. Research shows that staying healthy and fit is less expensive than paying for health-related expenses down the road. A 2009 study published in *The American Journal of Medicine* found that almost two-thirds of the U.S. bankruptcies had a health-related issue. The average out of pocket cost (that's after your insurance pays) for a hospital stay after a heart attack or stroke is about $20,000. That doesn't include the money you won't get paid for missing work or the inconvenience and burden you might put on your family, relatives, friends, or colleagues.

More than 70 percent of people hospitalized today are there because of food-related issues primarily from being overweight and obese. And most of it is preventable.

If you think eating healthy is expensive now, see how much it will cost if (or when) being overweight creates a health-related issue. Purchasing healthy foods and taking the time to prepare a healthy meal will seem cheap and less inconvenient than grabbing fast food now and paying to restore your health later.

Do you enjoy going out for dinner and drinking wine? Imagine how much money you could save if you ate out less often and drank less wine. There are many ways to reallocate food expenses in your budget. For example, frozen vegetables and fruit are usually as nutritious as their fresh counterparts so long as you don't microwave them.

Are you of the opinion that healthy food doesn't taste that good? Or, you don't like the taste of healthy foods? That's because your taste buds have been desensitized from eating too much deep-fried food loaded with salt and sugar. Be patient when switching to healthier whole foods. Here's a tip. Use healthy spices to boost the taste and flavor in your dishes. It will help re-train your taste buds. It goes without saying (but I'll say it anyway) that flavored salt is not a healthy spice. Read the labels of the bottles or canisters of seasoning compounds to see whether or how much salt is in them.

As you'll recall in a previous lesson, I explained that children eat too much-processed food loaded with high-fructose corn syrup or aspartame, sometimes both, so that fresh vegetables and fruits taste bitter and sour to them.

A myth that needs busting is that people need to exercise to lose weight. Exercise is important to staying fit and in shape. But exercise alone will not help you lose weight unless you can improve and modify your eating habits. Also, people tend to overestimate how many calories they burn exercising and underestimate how many calories they consume. If you exercise and fail to eat enough calories, your body will go into starvation mode and fight to retain weight. It's a delicate balance.

But you can lose weight simply by modifying and improving your eating habits and drinking more pure water. That does not translate into being fit. There is a difference. A person can look fit and trim, yet still be out of shape. You'll probably want to do both, but don't equate one with the other.

Probably your biggest challenge and obstacle for you is that you're just not motivated. There's a reason why it's easier for people to lose weight before a wedding or school reunion. But those types of motivators tend to be short-lived and fleeting much like a diet that is a temporary fix.

Do you still live in the past reminiscing about your glory days in high school or college when you were fit and trim? Do you share a cold beer remembering that high school or college football game you played? Stop looking in the rearview mirror of your life. My coach, Dick Woit, said, "Don't tell me what you did yesterday, show me what you can do today." There is nothing more damaging to your future potential to lose weight and keep it off than spending time dwelling on the past.

Do you share a cold beer remembering that high school or college football game you played? Your weight reflects your past eating habits. But it doesn't have to define what you choose to eat or drink today. Or what you'll weigh in the future by improving your eating and drinking habits. Learn from the past but don't let it pull you backward. Jim Rohn taught, "Let your past be a schoolmaster, not a club." Let your past instruct you, learn lessons from it, but don't allow it to continue to beat you down.

Do you make excuses for being overweight? Darren Hardy gave great advice: "Look back for lessons, not excuses." Do you make excuses for being overweight?

"Keep Moving Forward." Walt Disney

Have you attempted to lose weight in the past? Are you embarrassed that you failed? Many people attempt to reduce weight and repeatedly give up. And lots of them will beat themselves up for it. Instead of playing the blame game, use positive self-talk to support your weight-loss endeavor. Remember to use a food journal to record what you eat, where you eat, when you eat, and most importantly, why you're eating. Reviewing your habits and thinking about what you did right can keep you on the right track. And, if you've made a mistake, correct it and move forward. Avoid being harsh on yourself.

The goal is to eventually have an "ah-ha" moment to keep you motivated and focused.

Do you succumb to temptations such as office parties, birthday celebrations, or happy hour?

When this happens, be prepared. Remember the "if this happens, then I'll do this" scenario discussed in a previous lesson.

The purpose of this course is to help you make small, seemingly inconsequential adjustments and improvements to your daily eating routines so they become new habits that you do automatically without thinking. That way you won't need willpower or fear a lack of discipline.

Imagine attending a birthday celebration and without thinking just saying, "No thank you" when offered a piece of cake or a scoop of ice cream. Or, taking the piece of cake, having one bite and choosing not to eat the remainder. It can be done. I've done it, others are doing it, and you can do it too. Be patient.

Obstacles and challenges are made to overcome. Add the solutions you've been taught so far to your weight-reduction success arsenal. Be patient and you'll start to notice those unwanted and unhealthy pounds drop off, slow and steady; and stay off.

The simple formula to achieving a healthy weight and maintaining it:

- Eat holistic (whole) foods
- Mostly plants
- Not too much
- Avoid processed foods
- Drink lots of pure water
- Get adequate sleep

Are you frustrated because you're doing all the right things, you've lost a few pounds, but you hit the dreaded weight-loss plateau? That's mind-numbing and infuriating when you're putting forth effort and still not dropping pounds. Lighten up on yourself! Plateaus are very common. Don't give up. Your body hit a new weight "set point" and is adjusting.

Here are a few reasons you might hit a plateau or otherwise be struggling on your weight-reduction journey:

- You have an unrealistic weight-loss expectation. As you have learned in previous lessons, you didn't put all the weight on at once and you shouldn't expect to shed it all at once. Be patient. It's the small, seemingly inconsequential improvements to your eating habits, made consistently over a long time, that will give you noticeable results. The key words being "consistently" and "long-time."
- You're not eating enough nourishing food. Super-low calorie and elimination diets ignore the fact that food is fuel. You need to ingest enough nourishing foods to properly fuel your body. Otherwise, it will go into starvation mode and resist shedding the weight. Remember, it's more than just calories in and calories out. One hundred calories in a Hershey's chocolate bar is NOT the same one hundred calories of blueberries, spinach, mixed greens, or lean protein.
- You're not eating the right proportions of carbohydrates, protein, and good fats. For a healthy dietary intake, you need to eat a combination of healthy carbohydrates, proteins, and fats. This is one reason why you can lose weight on a keto diet, but it's not healthy nor sustainable.
- You're eating more than you think and you're not drinking as much water as you think. Solution? A food journal. When people track their food intake for the first time, they are usually shocked to see what and how much they have eaten throughout the day. Unless you're keeping track of how much water you're drinking, you might be shocked that it's not as much as you thought.
- Finally, you might not get enough "good" sleep. Without enough sleep, your body will not shed those unwanted pounds. The average person, without adequate sleep, will consume an extra 500 calories per day, usually from sugary junk food or caffeinated sodas in one day. You must reduce your caloric intake by 500 calories per day to lose one pound in a week. Without proper sleep, you might be going in the opposite direction without realizing it.

David Medansky

The average adult eating the Standard American Diet (SAD) consumes approximately 67 percent of their total caloric intake from just three foods – corn, soy, and wheat and their spinoffs and byproducts. A healthy amount of corn, soy, and wheat in the human diet should only be between 1 percent and 4 percent of the total daily calories. Yet, most Americans' calories come from corn, soy, and wheat products. And we wonder why there's an epidemic of overweight and obese people.

And, it's getting worse and will continue to get worse because most farm animals, such as cows, chickens, and hogs are fed corn and soy. These animals were meant to graze on grass, not corn and soy. Because of the economic advantages, farm-raised fish such as salmon, carp, and tilapia are being fed corn and soy. Fish are meant to eat a variety of things such as bugs, worms, and other smaller fish. This is one reason why eating farm-raised fish is unhealthy. There are numerous articles warning of the dangers of why eating farm-raised is bad for your health.

Here's the rub. People are consuming more than 67 percent of their daily caloric intake from corn, soy, and wheat, because of the chicken, beef and fish you're eating that's been fed these grains. Unless you're eating wild caught fish, grass-fed beef, or pastured raised chickens and eggs, you're being overloaded with corn, soy, and wheat from the food chain.

In a nutshell, farm-raised cows, chickens, and fish should be categorized as "processed" foods. Ponder this for a few minutes. Again, it's all about the food manufacturers bottom line. They do not care about your health or the health of their own families. It's about profit.

Chapter 12

Best Foods to Eat and Worst Foods to Avoid

You will never change your life until you change something you do daily. The secret of your [weight loss] success is found in your daily routine.
John Maxwell

If you are willing to do what others will not do, such as eat whole/holistic foods, avoid processed foods, including farm-raised beef, chickens, and fish, and drink pure water when others are not, then you will reduce your risk of suffering from chronic disease and illnesses and enjoy an energetic and vibrant life.

Until now you've learned mostly about the mental, emotional, and psychological aspects of reducing weight in a healthy and sustainable manner. In this chapter we will delve into the best foods to eat and what makes them so healthy as well as the worst foods to eat and the reasons you should avoid them.

Do you like nuts?

Hopefully, you're not allergic to all nuts, because there are many health benefits to eating certain raw, unprocessed, unsalted nuts and seeds. A 2018 study found that more than 81,000 people who consumed large amounts of meat protein experienced a 60 percent increase in cardiovascular disease, whereas those who consumed more nuts and seeds, about a hand-full of mixed nuts or seeds per day, decreased their risk of developing the same deadly heart problems by 40 percent. Because each of us has a different definition of what a handful means, a handful means approximately 7 to 8 nuts. This is also known as "the squirrel diet" – just kidding folks.

A 2017 study found that plant and animal protein are equally capable of building muscle, meaning lentils are just as good a protein as chicken. Or, if you're not a vegetarian, chicken is just as good of a protein as lentils.

Not every nut has the same nutritional benefits. According to Dr. David Freidman, New York Times best-selling author of *Food Sanity*, and Dana Hunnes, senior dietitian at the Ronald Reagan UCLA Medical Center, the nuts that are the best to eat are walnuts, chestnuts, pistachios, almonds, pecans, Brazil nuts, cashews, hazelnuts, macadamia nuts, and peanuts.

Walnuts. Walnuts are among the healthiest nuts because they contain the most antioxidants compared to any other nut and offer the healthiest kind of fat, omega 3 fatty acids. Omega 3 fatty acids prevent heart disease. Walnuts also contain iron (which supports oxygen-carrying red blood cells), selenium (which research shows may help prevent cancer), calcium, zinc, vitamin E, and some B-vitamins.

You can eat seven to nine walnuts a day. Eating too many walnuts can cause you to gain weight. Seven walnuts have about 90 calories.

Chestnuts. Chestnuts have the fewest calories at 55 per ounce. Walnuts have approximately 185 calories per ounce. But chestnuts have the least amount of protein and the most carbohydrates. Chestnuts also provide a respectable amount of manganese, which helps the body metabolize proteins and carbs. Research has found that the fiber found in chestnuts may aid in weight loss and weight management. Studies have found that chestnuts are good for heart health because of vitamin B12, vitamin B6, and Folate.

You should eat at most 3 ounces of chestnuts a day to maximize their benefits. Eating too many chestnuts can have unpleasant side effects such as the formation of air in the stomach (flatulence) and bloating.

Pistachios. These nuts are fun to eat and are great for stress eaters since they give your hands something to do. Pistachios are a great source of protein, fiber, antioxidants, and heart-healthy fats. They contain more vitamin B-6 than any other nut. B-6 is important for blood sugar regulation and the formation of hemoglobin.

Hemoglobin is a molecule that carries oxygen in red blood cells. Pistachios are rich in potassium. Potassium is important to support your muscles. An ounce of pistachios contains more potassium than half of a large banana. There are approximately 159 calories in one ounce of pistachios, which is about 49 kernels.

Nutritionists warn that eating too many pistachios may lead to excess weight.

Almonds. Almonds contain more fiber than any other nut, about 3 grams per nut. They also have the highest amount of vitamin E than any other nut. Almonds contain lots of healthy fats, protein, and magnesium. Magnesium helps to fight depression. Almonds have been shown to lower blood sugar levels, reduce blood pressure and lower cholesterol levels. Almonds are great to reduce weight because they help to reduce hunger. Who knew, almonds are a natural appetite suppressant? There are 160 calories in 23 almonds. I generally eat seven to nine almonds at one serving.

Pecans. Pecans have many vitamins, minerals, and antioxidants. They also contain monounsaturated fats, which help to improve cholesterol levels. Pecans provide more flavonoids than any other nuts. Flavonoids are anti-inflammatory antioxidants that help fight cardiovascular disease and the negative effects of aging. The downside of pecans is that they are high in calories, about 200 per ounce. They also have less protein than many other nuts. Ten pecan halves have about 98 calories.

Brazil Nuts. Brazil nuts are one of the best sources of selenium. Selenium is a mineral that's been proven to boost your immune system, improve your thyroid function, and might prevent cancer. Like pecans, brazil nuts are high in monounsaturated fat. They also are a good source of magnesium, zinc, calcium, vitamin E, and some B vitamins. Brazil nuts contain a high amount of ellagic acid. Ellagic acid inhibits blood flow and can reduce the growth of cancer cells. Aim to eat at least 1-2 raw brazil nuts per day because they contain a large amount of selenium. Too much selenium is detrimental to your health and may actually increase your risk for cancer. Each brazil nut has about 30 calories.

Cashews. Cashews have a lower fat content than most other nuts. Most of the fat in cashews is heart-healthy monosaturated fats, like those found in olive oil. They are a good source of magnesium, phosphorus, copper, and manganese. A study in the *Journal of Nutrition* shows cashews may help to reduce blood pressure and raise the "good" cholesterol levels. Each ounce of cashews has 163 calories, which is only 16 to 18 cashew nuts, so it's easy to eat multiple servings in one sitting if you aren't careful. You need to cut 500 calories out of your diet each day to lose one pound per week, and this will be hard to do if you eat too many servings of cashews, or combination of other nuts, in one day. Research also points to the benefits of cashews on your skin and hair, and even your nerves, due to their powerful micronutrient content.

Hazelnuts. Hazelnuts contain high amounts of phenolic compounds. Phenolic compounds are antioxidants that have been proven to decrease blood cholesterol and inflammation. They also help muscles and joints and aid in digestion. Ten hazelnuts have about 102 calories.

Macadamia Nuts. Macadamia nuts get a bad rap because they are high in fat. But 80 percent of the fat is monosaturated, the "good" fat. They're a good source of calcium, magnesium, and potassium. These three minerals help prevent bone loss. Ten to 12 macadamia nuts contain about 204 calories.

Peanuts. Peanuts are not a member of the nut family. They are legumes since they grow underground like beans. The nuts discussed in this lesson grow on trees and are considered tree nuts. Because so many people are allergic to peanuts, I'm not going to discuss them in this lesson.

Pay attention! This is important. Nutritionists recommend eating about an ounce or 28 grams of nuts per day. That's about as much as can fit in the palm of your hand. And they can be a mixture of nuts or a handful of one kind, like almonds. Most people tend to eat more than a handful of nuts in one sitting, let alone one day. Why is that a problem? Let's summarize:

- 10 macadamia nuts have 204 calories
- 10 hazelnuts have 102 calories
- 7 walnuts have about 90 calories

- 16 cashews have 163 calories
- 10 pecan halves have about 98 calories
- 23 almonds have about 160 calories
- 49 pistachios have approximately 159 calories

Let me see. If I add all those calories together, I'd consume 976 calories. If I top it off with just two Brazil nuts, I'd add 60 calories! All those nuts would be a whopping 1,036 calories. Wow! What does this mean to our diets? To lose weight without burning muscle mass, you need to consume between 1,250 and 1,500 calories per day. And the nuts are 1,036 calories. Imagine getting most of your calories from just nuts. That's why it's important to limit the total quantity of nuts you consume. One ounce of canned mixed nuts that are roasted and salted contains 813 calories. That's why it's extremely important to eat raw, unsalted nuts. Just because something might be healthy for you doesn't mean it won't cause you to gain weight.

What Are the Best Foods to Eat?

Avocado. The avocado is a rather unique fruit. It is botanically a large berry containing a single large seed. The seed is sometimes referred to as a pit. Numerous studies show that it has powerful health benefits. It is an incredibly popular food among health-conscious individuals and considered to be a superfood because of its numerous health benefits. The avocado's many health benefits are supported by scientific research. It contains a wide variety of nutrients, including 20 different vitamins and minerals. Some of the most abundant nutrients, in a single 3.5-ounce serving, include:

- Vitamin K
- Folate
- Vitamin C
- Potassium
- Vitamin B5
- Vitamin B6
- Vitamin E

It also contains small amounts of magnesium, manganese, copper, iron, zinc, phosphorous, and vitamins A, B1 (thiamine), B2 (riboflavin), and B3 (niacin).

An average-sized avocado has 160 calories, 2 grams of protein, and 15 grams of healthy fats. Although it contains 9 grams of carbs, 7 of those are fiber, so there are only 2 "net" carbs, making this a low-carb friendly plant food.

Avocados do not contain any cholesterol or sodium and are low in saturated fat. Avocados contain more potassium than bananas. Several studies show that having a high potassium intake is linked to reduced blood pressure, which is a major risk factor for heart attacks, strokes, and kidney failure.

Most of the fat in avocado is oleic acid, a monounsaturated fatty acid that is also the major component of olive oil. Oleic acid reduces inflammation and has been shown to have beneficial effects on genes linked to cancer.

Avocados are richer in dietary fiber than most other foods. Fiber is important for weight loss and metabolic health.

Heart disease is the most common cause of death in the world. Eight controlled studies showed that avocados can:

1. Reduce total cholesterol levels significantly.
2. Reduce blood triglycerides by up to 20 percent.
3. Lower LDL cholesterol by up to 22 percent.
4. Increase HDL (the "good") cholesterol by up to 11 percent.

This means that consistently eating avocados can reduce your risk of heart disease.

Avocados are high in nutrients that are extremely important for eye health. Studies show they drastically reduce the risk for cataract and macular degeneration, which are common in older adults.

Arthritis is a common problem in Western countries. Multiple studies suggest that avocado and soybean oil extracts — called avocado and soybean unsaponifiable — might reduce osteoarthritis.

Overall, there is some evidence that avocados are a weight-loss friendly food. In one study, people eating avocado with a meal felt 23 percent more satisfied and had a 28 percent lower desire to eat over the next 5 hours, compared to people who did not consume this fruit.

Including avocados in your diet may help you naturally eat fewer calories and make it easier for you to stick to healthy eating habits.

Apples. The old Welsh proverb "An apple a day keeps the doctor away" might be truer than you'd think. One of the most cultivated and consumed fruits in the world, apples continue to be praised as a "miracle food." A collection of research studies suggests that apples may well be one of the healthiest foods for you to include in your daily diet.

Apples contain thousands of phytonutrients, more than any other fruit. Phytonutrients help protect the body from the detrimental effects of free radicals. Research has shown that apples can improve neurological health. A 2006 study published in *Experimental Biology and Medicine* found that quercetin (an antioxidant abundantly found in apples) was one of two compounds that helped to reduce cellular death caused by oxidation and inflammation of the neurons. However, it should be noted that this study was funded by unrestricted grants provided by the U.S. Apple Association and Apple Products Research and Education Council.

A study published in the *Journal of Food Science* in 2008 suggested that eating apples may protect neuron cells against oxidative stress-induced neurotoxicity and reduce the risk of neurodegenerative disorders such as Alzheimer's disease.

Eating apples may reduce your risk of having a stroke. A study involving 9,208 men and women showed that those who ate the most apples over a 28-year period had the lowest risk for stroke.

Eating apples may lower your levels of bad cholesterol. A group of researchers at Florida State University found that older women who ate apples every day had 23 percent less bad cholesterol (LDL) and 4 percent more good cholesterol (HDL) after just six months.

Apples could also help lower your risk of diabetes. A study involving 187,382 people found that people who ate three servings of apples per week, or other fruits such as grapes, blueberries, raisins, or pears, had a 7 percent lower risk of developing Type 2 diabetes compared to those who did not.

According to Rui Hai Liu, a prominent researcher at Cornell, there is evidence suggesting that eating an apple a day may help prevent breast cancer. Liu said her research adds to "the growing evidence that increased consumption of fruits and vegetables, including apples, would provide consumers with more phenolics, which are proving to have important health benefits. I would encourage consumers to eat more and a wide variety of fruits and vegetables daily."

Apples are high in weight-loss friendly fiber. A medium-sized apple contains 4 grams of fiber. Eating fiber may slow the digestion of food and make you feel fuller with fewer calories. For this reason, foods high in fiber may help you eat fewer total calories overall, which helps you lose weight. With fewer than 100 calories in a medium-sized apple, apples are free of fat, sodium, and cholesterol. That same medium-sized apple contains 4 grams of dietary fiber, which is 17 percent of the recommended daily value for Americans.

Apples deserve to be called "nutritional powerhouses" because they contain thousands of phytonutrients as well as vitamin C, B-complex vitamins such as riboflavin, thiamin, and B-6, along with minerals such as calcium, potassium, and phosphorus.

Apple seeds contain cyanide, a powerful poison. Eating too many apple seeds can potentially be fatal. Don't eat the seeds!

Here are some fun facts about apples:

- There are 7,500 varieties, or cultivars, of apples grown throughout the world and 2,500 varieties in the U.S.
- The world's top apple producers are China, the United States, Turkey, Poland, and Italy.
- Apples are grown in all 50 states. As of 2010, the U.S. Department of Agriculture reported that 60 percent of the apples produced in the U.S. were grown in Washington state, 13 percent in New York, 6 percent in Michigan, 5 percent in Pennsylvania, 3 percent in California, and 2 percent in Virginia.
- In 1730, the first apple nursery was opened in Flushing, New York.
- The science of apple growing is called pomology.

- Apples are members of the rose family, Rosacea.

Be sure to eat the apple peels because the apple peels contain more antioxidant compounds, especially quercetin, and higher bioactivity than the apple flesh. Research showed that apples without the peels had less antioxidant activity than apples with the peels. Apples with the peels were also better able to inhibit cancer cell proliferation when compared to apples without the peels. More recent work has shown that apple peels contain anywhere from two to six times (depending on the variety) more phenolic compounds than in the flesh, and two to three times more flavonoids in the peels when compared to the flesh. The antioxidant activity of these peels was also much greater, ranging from two to six times greater in the peels when compared to the flesh, depending on the variety of the apple.

Berries. Berries are among the healthiest foods you can eat. They are delicious, nutritious and provide many impressive health benefits including:

- Berries may improve your blood sugar and insulin levels.
- They contain antioxidants. Antioxidants help fight inflammation.
- Berries are high in fiber. Fiber helps to decrease your appetite because it increases your feeling of fullness and reduces the number of calories your body absorbs from mixed meals.
- Berries are a heart-healthy food that may help lower cholesterol levels.
- Berries may help reduce skin wrinkling because the antioxidants in berries help control free radicals, one of the leading causes of skin damage that contributes to aging.

People who tend to eat at least three servings of berries per week see the most benefits.

Strawberries. Strawberries are a low-calorie food packed with vitamins, fiber, and particularly high levels of antioxidants known as polyphenols. They have no sodium, zero fat, and no cholesterol. They are among the top 20 fruits in antioxidant capacity and are a good source of manganese and potassium. Strawberries are an excellent source of vitamin C and manganese and contain a decent amount of folate (B9) and potassium. Strawberries have benefits for heart health and blood sugar control.

Strawberries are a healthy food to eat to lose weight because there are 49 calories in one cup of strawberries. One cup of whole strawberries contain about 8 large strawberries. The exciting research that is being done shows that the special nutritional components in strawberries might be able to stimulate your metabolism, help suppress your appetite, and control blood sugar.

Strawberries contain ellagic acid and anthocyanins which can assist with weight-loss in at least three ways:

1. Chronic inflammation blocks the hormones involved in keeping you lean. Anti-inflammatory foods like strawberries help restore normal function to weight-reducing hormones.
2. Anthocyanins increase the body's production of a hormone called adiponectin, which stimulates your metabolism and suppresses your appetite.
3. Both ellagic acid and anthocyanins slow the rate of digestion of starchy foods, controlling the rise in blood sugar that follows a starchy meal. This effect is used to control blood sugar in people with adult-onset Type 2 diabetes.

Blueberries. Blueberries are the fruits of a shrub that belong to the heath family, which includes the cranberry and bilberry as well as the azalea, mountain laurel, and rhododendron.

Blueberries can help you shed weight. Researchers studying blueberries found they have the potential to help reduce body fat. While blueberries have been well-documented for their cognitive and cardio-protective benefits, new research suggests that blueberries may change the way we metabolize fat and sugar. Blueberries are a source of fiber which has the power to fill you up and keep you full without consuming excess calories.

Recent study findings suggest that blueberries may influence genes which regulate fat-burning and storage, helping reduce abdominal fat and lower cholesterol. When combined with a low-fat diet, blueberries might also lower triglycerides and improve blood sugar levels, each benefits of a comprehensive weight-loss plan. A 1/2-cup serving of fresh blueberries has approximately 42 calories. One pint of blueberries should fill about two dry cups which is about four servings.

For a sweet treat at the end of dinner or a healthy snack, nibble on frozen blueberries. The cold transforms the berries into a sorbet-like texture that will quell your craving for ice cream.

Raspberries. Raspberries remain one of the world's most consumed berries. They can range in color from the popular red and black varieties to purple, yellow, or golden. Each color berry has a unique composition of vitamins, minerals, and antioxidants.

Raspberries have a high polyphenol content which may reduce the risk of cardiovascular disease by preventing platelet buildup and reducing blood pressure via anti-inflammatory mechanisms.

Aedin Cassidy, Ph.D., a nutrition professor at Norwich Medical School at the University of East Anglia in the United Kingdom, led an 18-year study with Harvard Public School of Health that tracked 93,600 women aged 25-42 years. She states that their study was able to show "for the first time that a regular, sustained intake of anthocyanins from berries can reduce the risk of a heart attack by 32 percent in young and middle-aged women."

One-half cup of raspberries has about as much potassium, approximately 200mg, as a small apple or medium size peach.

The fiber and water content in raspberries help to prevent constipation and maintain a healthy digestive tract. Increased fiber intake has also been shown to lower blood pressure and cholesterol levels and enhance weight loss for obese individuals.

One cup of raspberries, about 36 to 38 berries, contains 64 calories. Raspberries also contain the antioxidants alpha and beta-carotene, lutein, zeaxanthin, and choline. Raspberries are also a good source of polyphenols. Studies show polyphenols may prevent or reduce the risk of chronic diseases including cancer and heart disease.

Blackberries. A one-cup serving of fresh blackberries contains slightly more than 60 calories. Nearly 90 percent of the calories come from carbohydrates. This serving of blackberries has a little less than 14 grams of carbohydrates, amounting to 55 calories from carbs. Don't let the carb content of blackberries scare you off because healthy carbs, such as those in blackberries, are your body's main energy source.

Fiber has a recommendation separate from carbohydrates. According to the Centers for Disease Control and Prevention, based on a 1,500-calorie diet, you need 21 grams of fiber each day. One cup of blackberries amounts to 35 percent of your total fiber needs for the entire day.

Because blackberries help fill you up and are low in calories, they are excellent for any healthy weight-loss meal plan. Blackberries, however, lack some essential nutrients so don't overindulge in blackberries during your weight-loss journey. If you overindulge eating blackberries you may be getting too little protein or healthy fat in your weight-loss diet. Therefore, it is important to eat blackberries in moderation.

Here are some other tips to help increase your berry consumption:
- Always keep a bag of frozen berries on hand for adding to smoothies and oatmeal
- Forgo the syrupy sweetness of canned fruit cocktail and make your own fresh fruit cocktail with raspberries, pineapple, sliced peaches, and strawberries
- Add berries and walnuts to your chicken salad
- Add berries to plain Greek yogurt with a drizzle of agave nectar and sliced almonds.
- Top whole grain waffles or pancakes with fresh berries.
- Blend various berries separately in a food processor with a little water and use as a fresh syrup to top desserts or breakfast foods
- Mix berries into a spinach salad with walnuts and goat cheese.

Pastured Eggs. What are "pastured eggs"? There is no legal definition of pastured chickens, however, the Humane Farm Animal Care (HFAC), a non-profit certification organization, has set the standard for eggs labeled "pastured." Pastured eggs come from chickens that are free to wander outdoors in a pasture where they can eat grass, worms, bugs, and whatever else pleases their palate. The eggs these hens lay are now available in some supermarkets and specialty stores. They are usually costlier than organic eggs, ranging in price from about $5 to $9 a dozen.

Are you wondering, if they worth the added cost?

Whether pastured eggs are worth the higher cost depends on whether you think they are better than eggs from chickens raised in factory settings. Here's some more information to help you decide.

To meet the HFAC standard and earn the "certified humane" designation, egg producers must show that hens are outdoors year-round with access to housing where they can go at night to protect themselves from predators. The organization also mandates that producers allot 2.5 acres per 1,000 birds and rotate the fields. To the best of my research, only three "pasture raised" egg companies and one "free range" company have earned HFAC's "certified humane" label.

You might think that the same general principles apply to "free-range" hens, but while that phrase may suggest happy chickens wandering around a barnyard or field, the reality is that most live in huge industrial aviaries with, on average, one square foot of space apiece (although a new California law requires that chickens be given enough space to extend their limbs and turn around freely).

Legally, the term "free-range" means that hens have "access" to the outdoors, but in practice that access usually amounts to not much more than a few small doors – comparable to a cat door – that allow the hens to get out onto a screened porch where some grass may or may not grow. Most of the birds never go outside.

Sadly, an estimated 95 percent of eggs in the U.S. come from chickens raised in cages that house from four to 12 birds, giving each bird roughly 67 square inches of floor space (about the size of an iPad).

Organic eggs come from "free-range" chickens that mostly live in large, crowded aviaries with limited outdoor access. Legally, to qualify as organic, eggs must come from chickens raised on organic (no pesticides) feed. Pastured eggs aren't considered organic.

As for nutritional value, some evidence suggests that pastured eggs may be better for you. A 2010 study from Penn State showed that they had twice as much vitamin E and long-chain omega-3 fatty acids as eggs from caged hens.

Don't confuse "pastured" with "pasteurized," which designates eggs that have been heated to just below the coagulation point to destroy pathogens. These are sometimes available in grocery stores, but most are used in commercially prepared foods.

Green Leafy Vegetables. Salads are a great way to pack in the nutrients without packing on the pounds. The best salads contain a rainbow of vitamin-rich veggies, dark leafy greens, metabolism-boosting lean protein, non-starchy carbs, and a dose of healthy fat. Salads, however, too often fall short of being a healthy meal because of the salad dressing added and the most basic ingredient is lettuce. Since the greens are the foundation for the salad, it's important to build a better one by choosing the best-mixed greens.

Dark leafy greens — like spinach, arugula, kale, turnip greens, and so many more — have countless health benefits. They play a significant role in decreasing our risk of diabetes because of their fiber and magnesium content, which in turn helps your metabolism and overall nerve and muscle function. The high levels of iron in spinach and Swiss chard are great for bringing oxygen to your muscles, and kale is loaded with vitamin C and calcium. Dark leafy greens, in general, help to prevent system-wide inflammation, reducing arthritis pain and blood clotting. Bonus: They even contain a very small amount of omega-3 fats.

Leafy green vegetables are an important part of a healthy diet. They're packed with vitamins, minerals, and fiber but are low in calories. Eating a diet rich in leafy greens can offer numerous health benefits including reduced risk of obesity, heart disease, high blood pressure, and mental decline.

The Bottom Line: Leafy greens are great for you, and you should be eating more of them! Skip the iceberg and other light-colored lettuces and instead load up on kale, spinach, romaine, arugula, and other dark greens.

Cabbage comes in green, white, and purple colors. It belongs to the *Brassica* family, along with Brussels sprouts, kale, and broccoli.

Iceberg lettuce has very little nutritional value and doesn't do much for your body. It's made up of 95 percent water and contains only small amounts of fiber and minerals. So, while iceberg lettuce is low in calories and is not bad for you, it's not that good either.

Raw Cheese. Raw, or unpasteurized, milk has been a controversial topic for quite some time, with strong arguments on each side. But with the FDA's increased inspections on raw milk cheese, the debate has picked up new steam. Some believe it's the agency's first step toward changing current regulations or even banning raw milk cheese altogether.

Of course, these are the same folks who approve aspartame and high-fructose corn syrup to be added to your food. Oh, and let's not forget the scientifically engineered fat and cholesterol substitute Olean.

Healthy organic, raw milk is beneficial to your health, adds good bacteria into your gut, and brings its own package of digestive enzymes with it. Raw cheese abounds in enzymes that help to digest the fats and proteins. When the food you eat has abundant bacteria and enzymes, then the digestive system is not overtaxed. Most people suffer from depleted digestive enzymes and your health is often compromised for it. People often complain about feeling sluggish and lacking energy. This is because they are chronically short on healthy gut flora and digestive enzymes, as the food we eat is mostly "dead."

Raw cheese from 100% grass-fed cows is healthier. Why grass-fed? Grass-fed cows contain an average of two to three times more Conjugated Linoleic Acid (CLA) than grain-fed cows. CLA is a compound that used to be in foods with healthy fat before the advent of the modern low-fat diet. Now science is indicating that one side effect of people cutting out fat is cutting out CLA, a component of fat that has been shown to slow the process of some types of cancer and heart disease. It also appears to help reduce body fat and increase lean muscle mass. CLA is a fatty acid that occurs naturally in many foods and is especially high in milk and meat from ruminant animals such as cows, sheep, and goats. CLA is produced by bacteria in the rumen, the first stomach of a cow, which receives food or cud from the esophagus, partly digests it with the aid of bacteria, and passes it to the reticulum. This is because grain-based diets reduce the pH of the digestive system in ruminant animals, which inhibits the growth of the bacterium that produces CLA.

Grass-fed also means that the cows never receive grain at any given time. Grass-fed cows are on pasture 100 percent of the time or feeding on stored grass baleage or dry hay when inside for milking or bad weather.

Worst Foods to Eat

Anything with high-fructose corn syrup. You hear about high-fructose corn syrup, or HFCS, all the time. But do you know what the ingredient is, or how it affects your health? High-fructose corn syrup (HFCS) is a type of artificial sugar made from corn syrup.

HFCS is commonly found in sodas, desserts, and certain breakfast cereals. It is often criticized for its contribution to America's obesity epidemic. It's also been linked with chronic conditions such as Type 2 diabetes, heart disease, and even some cancers.

The sweetener is made from processed corn starch. Starches are made of long chains of linked sugars, and HFCS is produced by breaking down the starch into a syrup made of the sugar glucose. Manufacturers then add enzymes to the substance to convert some of the glucose into fructose, which tastes much sweeter.

So, why don't brands just use regular table sugar? Because HFCS is much cheaper, hence why it became so popular starting in the 1970s. But the affordable ingredient also comes with a catch. Studies have shown that animals who eat a diet high in HFCS gain more weight than those who don't. Even worse, the ingredient doesn't fill them up, so it makes them more likely to overeat.

The corn industry spends millions on misinformation campaigns to convince consumers and health care professionals of the safety of their product. But, HFCS and cane sugar are NOT biochemically identical or processed the same way by the body. High-fructose corn syrup is an industrial food product and far from "natural" or a naturally occurring substance. It is extracted from corn stalks through a process so secret that Archer Daniels Midland and Carghill would not allow the investigative journalist Michael Pollan to observe it for his book *The Omnivore's Dilemma*. The sugars are extracted through a chemical enzymatic process resulting in a chemically and biologically novel compound called HFCS. Some basic biochemistry will help you understand this. Regular cane sugar (sucrose) is made of two-sugar molecules bound tightly together– glucose and fructose in equal amounts. The enzymes in your digestive tract must break down the sucrose into glucose and fructose, which are then absorbed into the body. HFCS also consists of glucose and fructose, not in a 50-50 ratio, but a 55-45 fructose-to-glucose ratio in an unbound form. Fructose is sweeter than glucose.

And HFCS is cheaper than sugar because of the government farm bill corn subsidies. Products with HFCS are sweeter and cheaper than products made with cane sugar. This allowed the average soda size to balloon from 8 ounces to 20 ounces with little financial costs to manufacturers but great human costs of increased obesity, diabetes, and chronic disease.

Back to biochemistry. Since there is no chemical bond between them, no extra digestion is required so they are more rapidly absorbed into your bloodstream. Fructose goes right to the liver and triggers *lipogenesis* (the production of fats like triglycerides and cholesterol). This is the reason it is the major cause of liver damage in this country and causes a condition called "fatty liver" which affects 70 million people.

Rapidly absorbed glucose triggers big spikes in insulin–your body's major fat storage hormone. Both these features of HFCS lead to increased metabolic disturbances that drive increases in appetite, weight gain, diabetes, heart disease, cancer, dementia, and more.

The top 10 foods with the highest amount of High-fructose corn syrup are:

1. Some yogurts
2. Most bread
3. Many frozen pizzas
4. Cereal bars
5. Cocktail peanuts
6. Boxed mac & cheese
7. Most salad dressings
8. Tomato-based sauces
9. Applesauce
10. Canned fruit

Avoid all processed food with Olean. In recent years, many types of "fat-free" foods have come into the marketplace. One such type of these foods contain artificial fats that are substituted for the natural fats and oils found in the foods. These artificial fats add no fat or calories to the diet because they are not digested or absorbed by the body. The main artificial fat commercially in use is Olestra. Olestra is marketed under the name Olean by Proctor and Gamble, Inc.

Unfortunately, Olean may not be as healthy as it first sounds. It has been shown to cause gastrointestinal symptoms including abdominal discomfort, flatulence, and changes in stool consistency. More importantly, it interferes with the absorption of fat-soluble vitamins from food when present in the small intestine at the same time as other foods. Because it is nonpolar, Olean can dissolve fat-soluble vitamins. Hence, Olean in the small intestine competes with fat-containing micelles in the intestine for absorption of fat-soluble vitamins. Anything the Olean absorbs is carried out of the body with it and is therefore not available for absorption by the body. Olean is banned in China, the U.K., and Canada. Olean/Olestra is used in the preparation of most snacks. Some snacks that have olestra as an ingredient:

1. Doritos
2. Frito Lay
3. Potato chips
4. Fat-free Pringles

5. Fat-free Ritz and Wheat Thins

Avoid diet sodas because they contain aspartame. Aspartame is an artificial sugar substitute. It has 92 known adverse side effects! Including weight gain.

A 25-year study found that moderate consumption of aspartame is linked to a 65 percent higher likelihood of being overweight and a 41 percent increased likelihood of being obese.

Although aspartame is approved by the Food and Drug Administration and the European Food Safety Authority, the consumer advocate organization Center for Science in the Public Interest has cited numerous studies that suggest problems with the sweetener, including a study by the Harvard School of Public Health. Yet, if you do research on aspartame, you'll find evidence that there's no consensus as to whether aspartame is "bad" for you.

Aspartame is one of the most common artificial sweeteners in use today. It is made by joining together the amino acids aspartic acid and phenylalanine. Amino acids are the building blocks of proteins and are found naturally in many foods. Aspartame is used in many foods and beverages because it is about 200 times sweeter than sugar, so much less of it can be used to give the same level of sweetness. This, in turn, lowers the calories in the food or beverage.

Research shows that aspartame does not help people lose weight and that it is associated with weight gain. Sounds counterintuitive, right? It's obviously not about the calories, because diet beverages with aspartame have no calories. One study suggests aspartame blocks an enzyme that prevents obesity. Other research has found that aspartame can alter how we process fat – obviously not in a good way. And aspartame may stimulate our appetites, and that leads to eating more. One thing the studies agree on: more research is needed on this entirely fake food.

As of 2014, aspartame was the largest source of methanol in the American diet.

Methanol is toxic in large quantities, yet smaller amounts may also be concerning when combined with free methanol because of enhanced absorption. Free methanol is present in some foods and is also created when aspartame is heated. Free methanol consumed regularly may be a problem because it breaks down into formaldehyde, a known carcinogen, and neurotoxin, in the body. As stated earlier, aspartame was created in 1965 by Searle & Company. Searle was purchased by Monsanto in 1985. Monsanto manufacturers DDT, Agent Orange, and GMOs.

Roaches and ants won't eat it. Cats and dogs won't eat it. House flies won't eat it. But, the FDA (Food and Drug Administration) says aspartame is safe for *YOU*.

Orange juice and fruit juices. Fruits are incredibly nutrient-dense and full of vitamins, minerals, and fiber, but they contain few calories, making them good for weight loss. Also, its high fiber and water contents make it very filling and appetite-suppressing. But try sticking to whole fruits instead of fruit juice. There's a big difference between the health effects of fruit and those of fruit juice because while whole fruit is low in calories and a good source of fiber, the same is not necessarily true of fruit juice.

In the process of juice-making, the juice is extracted from the fruit, removing its beneficial fiber and providing a concentrated dose of calories and sugar. Oranges are one great example. One small orange contains 45 calories and 9 grams of sugar, while one cup of orange juice contains 134 calories and 23 grams of sugar. The sugar content of fruit juice is actually like sugar-sweetened beverages like Coca Cola. So, eat the whole fruit, but avoid fruit juice if you're trying to lose weight.

Bananas. There is a dispute among nutritionist, dieticians, and other health experts over whether bananas are good or bad to eat if trying to lose weight. Bananas are high in many nutrients and provide many health benefits. They contain lots of fiber, carbs, and some essential vitamins and minerals. A medium-sized banana contains:

- Potassium
- Vitamin B6
- Vitamin C
- Magnesium
- Copper
- Manganese

- Fiber

Bananas contain around 105 calories, of which 90 percent come from carbs. Most of the carbohydrates in ripe bananas are sugars — sucrose, glucose, and fructose. On the other hand, bananas are low in both fat and protein. Unripe, green bananas are high in starch and resistant starch, while ripe, yellow bananas contain mostly sugars. Filling up on high fiber, low-calorie snacks can help with weight loss and weight maintenance.

These foods help prevent feelings of hunger and subsequent overeating, without adding lots of unnecessary calories to your diet. In fact, bananas could help fill you up a lot better than other higher-calorie snacks. However, they aren't quite as filling as some other fruits. For example, apples and oranges are more filling than bananas, calorie per calorie.

Chapter 13

Fasting

You can't go back and change the beginning, but you can start where you are and change the ending.
C.S. Lewis

In this chapter, we will delve into the ancient practice of fasting that dates to the beginning of mankind when our bodies were forced to adapt to times of famine and food scarcity. It still costs nothing to practice and could transform the health of every cell in your body!

The information on fasting is presented for educational purposes only and is not designed to treat or cure any health conditions. If you want to incorporate fasting strategies into your weight-loss journey, please consult with your medical doctor or qualified health practitioner first to make sure it is OK for your unique health situation and/or condition.

There are some people who should NOT fast. These include, but are not limited to, pregnant women, newborn babies, young children, high-level athletes who do intense training, individuals with a history of eating disorders, Type 1 diabetics, and individuals with pathological cachexia. (Cachexia is a condition that causes extreme weight loss and muscle wasting. It is a symptom of many chronic conditions, such as cancer, chronic renal failure, HIV, and multiple sclerosis.)

So, what about fasting? How many of you are seeing ads and online messages about intermittent fasting? With all the hype about it, you may feel it's just another modern diet fad. The truth is, fasting is thousands of years old.

Fasting is one of the most ancient and widespread healing traditions in the world. Hippocrates, who is widely considered the father of modern medicine, prescribed the practice of fasting and the consumption of apple cider vinegar as treatments. Hippocrates wrote, "To eat when you are sick, is to feed your illness."

The ancient Greeks had a lot to say about fasting. Writer and historian Plutarch wrote, "Instead of using medicine, better fast today." Plato said, "I fast for greater physical and mental efficiency." Aristotle, his pupil, also fasted. According to Paracelsus, one of the three fathers of Western medicine, "Fasting is the greatest remedy–the physician within."

Whenever fasting is mentioned, there is always the same eye-rolling response. Starvation. Can you relate to this? Did you roll your eyes, too?

Fasting is not starvation. Starvation is the *involuntary* absence of food. It is neither deliberate nor controlled. Starving people have no idea when and where their next meal will come from.

Fasting is the *voluntary* withholding of food for spiritual, health, or other reasons. The two terms, "starvation" and "fasting," should never be confused with each other. In a sense, fasting is part of everyday life. The term 'break-fast' is the meal that breaks the fast, which, for many people, is done daily.

Fasting isn't abnormal. It's a natural healing process. Some call it a natural healing process, a way to get back to normal. Fasting is widespread. Fasting remains part of virtually every major religion in the world. Jesus Christ, Buddha, and the prophet Muhammed all shared a common belief in the power of fasting for cleansing or purification. In other words, healing.

The practice of fasting varies between cultures and religions. In Buddhism, food is often consumed only in the morning, and followers fast from noon until the next morning daily. In addition to this, there may be various water-only fasts for days or weeks on end. Greek Orthodox Christians may follow various fasts over 180-200 days of the year. Crete is considered the poster child of the healthy Mediterranean diet. Yet most of the population of Crete followed the Greek Orthodox tradition of fasting. Muslims fast from sunrise to sunset during the holy month of Ramadan.

It's only until recently in human history that people have not gone for extended periods of time without food. Throughout our evolutionary history, there would be periods lasting days, weeks, or months during which food resources were scarce.

Today, in our modern society, we are blessed, or cursed depending on the source, with an abundance of food. Unfortunately, much of our food today is processed. We eat foods full of sugar, dairy, and grains that are high in calories and unhealthy fats. Worse, our bodies do not get enough nutrients. Yet we overconsume.

Most people are overconsuming grain. When you eat too much grain, you overconsume Omega-6. Too much Omega-6 causes inflammation to your body. Dr. Lori Shemek wrote about this in her best-selling book, *FATflammation!* Grains are in virtually all processed foods. The Food Pyramid in the U.S. is a solid base of grain. Also, you're probably eating a lot of processed sugar made from grains – specifically corn – without realizing it. And this causes inflammation in your body.

Dr. Peter Osborne, the clinical director at the Origins Healthcare in Sugarland, Texas, and author of the best-selling book *No Grain, No Pain,* provides a great analogy. Dr. Osborne says to imagine that you go home from work every day and prepare your meals, eat, but never do your dishes. The dishes keep piling up in the sink. Eventually, they start spilling out of the sink and onto the countertop. Before you know it, you have bugs eating the debris of the food left on the dishes. And you have a huge mess in your house because you didn't do the dishes.

Dr. Osborne says that's what happens in your stomach. When you put too much in and don't have normal "housekeeping," the stomach becomes overwhelmed and your gastrointestinal system becomes a breeding ground for bacteria. And when you eat all the time and don't give your stomach a rest, it becomes exhausted. Your gut needs a vacation!

This where fasting comes in. You're giving your body a chance to clean the dishes, so to speak. It gives your body a chance to rest and repair itself.

My friend Dr. Rachel Smartt told me another analogy to explain the importance of fasting. Dr. Smartt described fasting as your body being a power lawnmower and the food you consume being wet grass. As you mow wet grass, it sticks to the undercarriage and begins to clog the mower's blade. To keep the mower's engine from overheating, you must clean the undercarriage and remove the wet grass. Otherwise, the accumulation of the wet grass will make the engine work harder and eventually cause it to burn out. This is what happens when you put too much food into your system. Fasting gives your body time to cleanse itself. If you don't allow your body time to clean itself, it will put a strain on your digestive system and other organs. Dr. Bob Martin, Certified Clinical Nutritionist (C.C.N.), host of "The Dr. Bob Martin Show," the largest syndicated alternative health show in the U.S., said, "If you wear out your body where are you going to live?"

There are many types of fasts. For instance, there is intermittent fasting, water fast, a bone broth fast, a green juice fast, liquid nutrition fast, and fasting mimicking diet, to mention just a few. Because this can become a very confusing topic, this lesson will be limited to intermittent and extended fasting.

There is a difference between intermittent fasting and extended fasting or long fasting. If you decide to do an extended fast, it MUST be under the supervision of a medical doctor or qualified health professional. Please, do NOT do an extended fast without proper medical supervision.

What Happens to Your Body When You Fast?

When you fast intermittently, insulin levels go down and glucagon goes up which has been shown to have benefits such as increased metabolism, more energy, improved mood, and weight loss.

Fasting can also increase the diversity of bacteria in your gut, which is important for your immune system and overall health. Researchers have linked daily fasting to activation of the gene that strengthens the gut barrier to protect us from harmful microbes, contaminants, and other substances that can trigger immune reactions.

How and When Do You Fast?

Intermittent fasting, also called "time-restricted feeding," is the practice of eating food within a certain time period during the day.

Intermittent fasts can last as little as four hours or as long as 36 hours. Anything longer than 36 hours is considered an extended fast and MUST be done under the supervision of a medical doctor or qualified health professional.

For those of you who've never done an intermittent fast, begin with one of the most common approaches to intermittent fasting: eat your meals within an eight-hour period and avoid food, except pure water, during the next 16 hours. Why 16 hours? Some research suggests that 16 hours is the optimal amount of time for creating the caloric restriction that happens during fasting and to give your cells time to cleanse themselves. Make certain you drink between eight and 16 ounces of water when you first wake up. This will help reduce morning hunger and prolong the fast and improve the cleansing process.

"The Best of all Medicines is Resting and Fasting." Benjamin Franklin

This is what an intermittent fast could look like: You finish dinner at 7:00 p.m. and you don't eat again until 7:00 a.m. That's it! That is a 12-hour intermittent fast.

This is really the easiest way to start any kind of fasting. You might already be implementing this into your weight-reduction journey without realizing it.

According to Dr. David Friedman, author of the New York Times bestselling book *Food Sanity*, breakfast is the most important meal of the day. Dr. Friedman said, "I fast for 13 hours every day from 8 p.m. until 9 a.m. That's six-plus months out of the year that I spend fasting. Then I break my fast each morning with a healthy 'break-fast' (the true meaning of the word.) This gives me the stamina I need to do my physical job before having a small lunch. So many chronically overweight patients skip breakfast each day and eat a large lunch instead. I believe what you eat is more important than when you eat."

Dr. David Jonkers, a doctor of natural medicine and corrective care chiropractor, refers to this type of fast as a brunch fast because you're eating breakfast a few hours later than most.

Jon Gabriel, in his 12-week Total Transformation Experience program, refers to fasting as shifting your hunger habits. According to Gabriel, "… the best chance you have of burning fat is when you've gone 14 or more hours without eating. If you can go 16 or even 18 hours without eating, your body is going to be full-on burning fat."

Jon Gabriel said he prefers to eat his food between 10:00 a.m. and 4:00 p.m. This is referred to as a "Strong Fast." Gabriel explains the reasons for that is because his body has gotten into the habit of eating at that time. He suggests that you can change the time period to range between 11:00 a.m. and 5:00 p.m. or 12 noon and 6:00 or 8:00 p.m. in the evening.

Gabriel is realistic. He understands that there will be times when you're going out with friends for dinner or attending other events that might include dinner or other foods. According to Gabriel, "Don't worry about it."

You don't need to make a religion out of intermittent fasting. It is not a hard and fast rule. You don't need to do intermittent fasting every day. These are just guidelines to shift your hunger habit. Experts have their own views and opinions about what is the best way to do intermittent fasting, whether it is 12, 13, 16, or 18 hours. You need to figure out and determine what is best for you. If you work the night shift or wake up at different hours, make your own fasting schedule. The concept is that you're eating most of your food during a six- to eight-hour period and you're doing it when your body has adapted to the process. Go at your own pace. You don't want to force your body into an intermittent fasting regimen if it's not ready.

Here's another thought: Don't force yourself into eating during only a six to eight-hour window of time if you're hungry the rest of the time. Intermittent fasting is not right for you at this moment. That doesn't mean you won't be able to do this in the future. Make small adjustments to your daily eating routine consistently over a long period of time until it becomes your habit.

There's a difference between being a perfectionist when it comes to intermittent fasting and seeking excellence. There is a

Vince Lombardi quote even for this: "Perfection is not attainable, but if we chase perfection, we can catch excellence."

Even though intermittent fasting has many benefits to help heal your body, it doesn't mean you can eat anything you want such as processed foods and junk food, and it doesn't mean you can eat as much as you want. You still need to eat whole (holistic) foods and watch your portion sizes. If you keep eating 2,000 calories a day or more, you're not going to shed those extra pounds. One caveat, if you're doing intensive exercise or heavy physical activity, you'll need to adjust your caloric intake to a higher amount to make sure you don't put your body into starvation mode.

100 Percent Natural Cellular Detox

Are you familiar with the term autophagy? (Pronounced "aw-TOFF-uh-gee.") The most basic definition of autophagy is to think of it as your body's own cellular detox program. But unlike trendy "cleanses" and "detoxes," autophagy is 100 percent physiological. Fasting advocates say autophagy allows your own biology to restore vitality, slow down the aging process, prevent disease, and help you bust through a weight-loss plateau.

What this means for you is this type of cleanse doesn't involve drinking any weird beverages, eating tasteless cardboard-like food, or torturing yourself with hours of excessive exercise. Autophagy is completely natural and happening inside of you all the time to different degrees, even when you don't realize it. It's as natural for our cells to self-cleanse (autophagy literally means self ["auto"] – eating ["phagy"]) as it is for them to undergo normal wear and tear.

Healthy, intermittent fasting can activate autophagy. Now you have a less-complicated anti-aging strategy that can increase cellular repair and renewal every day. That's the idea advanced by Japanese cell biologist Yoshinori Ohsumi, who won the Nobel Prize in Medicine in 2016 for his research on autophagy. Ohsumi proved autophagy to be the one true physiological detox program that is 100 percent backed by science.

Persistent Myths About Fasting – They're Wrong

Let's take a minute and look at a couple of persistent myths about fasting. One is that fasting shuts down the thyroid gland in women. Thomas Delauer, a celebrity trainer and author of the book, *Top Ten Intermittent Fasting Hacks: Ten Key Tips to Make Fasting Easier & More Effective* said that is just misinformation. He doesn't know where that misinformation comes from.

The other myth about fasting is that it slows your metabolism and forces the body into starvation mode, causing the body to retain fat. A review of more than 30 independent studies demonstrates that the opposite is true. The studies indicate that intermittent fasting can accelerate and enhance weight loss. The studies found that intermittent fasters shed an average of seven to 11 pounds during a 10-week period.

Here's a summary of the benefits of fasting gleaned from various books and articles on the topic:

- **It improves energy levels.** People who regularly practice intermittent fasting have noticed improved energy levels.
- **It reduces inflammation**. Numerous studies have shown that fasting reduces the number of inflammatory cytokines produced in your body.
- **It stimulates fat burning**.
- **It takes the stress off your digestive system**. Digestion is a stressful and demanding process on the body. You can reduce the stress level of your digestive tract by fasting and allowing it to heal and repair itself.
- **It stimulates cellular autophagy**.
- **It improves genetic repair processes**. Research has shown that cells have a greater lifespan during times of famine and food scarcity. Fasting enhances cellular rejuvenation by acting on certain genetic repair processes.
- **It can help improve insulin sensitivity**. Insulin, which is a hormone, helps your body burn sugar for fuel. Improved insulin sensitivity helps people with insulin resistance and Type 2 diabetes.

- **It can help reduce your risk for chronic disease**. All chronic diseases are caused by chronic inflammation. Fasting is the most powerful nutritional method to reduce inflammation in your body.

  When you reduce your inflammatory levels, you influence your genes to induce better health for all your organs, systems, tissues, and the cells of your body. Doing this will greatly reduce your risk of chronic disease and acts as an anti-aging mechanism.

  Most people shouldn't need to purchase products that claim to reduce inflammation if you are in the habit of intermittent fasting at least three times per week. **I don't mean medicine: Always consult with your medical doctor or qualified health professional before stopping any anti-inflammatory medication you are currently prescribed.**

- **It can help you improve your food choices**. Many of you might be struggling with mindless eating and have struggled with sugar, carbs, dairy, and other cravings. Fasting can help you realize that these cravings are mental and emotional and that you can overcome them.

- **It can help improve your mood**. Fasting elevates your ketone levels. When this happens, many people experience improvement in their mood, have higher mental clarity and creativity. Usually achieving this improvement requires an extended fast of three to four days.

The Ketogenic Diet

As long as I mentioned ketones, let's talk about the ketogenic diet for a minute. The ketogenic diet is among the widely talked about and debated diet trends today. Science backs up the ketogenic diet as having numerous health benefits. When done properly, it can help reduce the risk of heart disease, improve glycemic control in both Type 1 and Type 2 diabetes, help people reduce weight, and improve neurological disorders such as Parkinson's and epilepsy. The key is that the ketogenic diet must be conducted properly.

The ketogenic diet is not new. It supposedly resembles the way people ate before humanity developed agriculture and enabled the domestication of staple crops such as wheat and corn. Before this huge shift in diet, people ate a variety of wild plants and animals and far fewer carbohydrates or sugar. Their diet was naturally low in carbohydrates and forced them to burn fat for fuel as opposed to carbs. This is the core of the ketogenic diet – burning fat instead of carbohydrates.

The primary focus of the keto diet is to force the body into a state of ketosis, where metabolism shifts from burning carbohydrates as the primary energy or fuel source to using fat, or "ketones bodies." Ketones are a special type of fat that acts as a cellular super fuel. To achieve ketosis, you must consume a diet high in healthy fat (the operative word being "healthy") and significantly lower your intake of sugar and carbohydrates. This allows the blood sugar level to drop so that glucose is dramatically less available to the body to burn as fuel. In the absence of glucose, your body will use ketones for energy. Ketosis burns fat, which assists with weight loss and transitions the body to use a better fuel source.

An indelicate word of warning: Many people incorrectly eliminate all carbs from their diet. This is not healthy because it reduces your dietary fiber intake. When you consume too little dietary fiber, you develop constipation. Constipation is very common for those who eat too little healthy dietary fiber. If you attempted a keto type diet, can you relate to this?

Another drawback to improperly adhering to a ketogenic diet is not getting enough nutrition from a variety of foods that your body requires to maintain good health.

One of the most powerful tools a person on the ketogenic diet can use is intermittent fasting. Intermittent fasting reduces calories, which then requires the body to burn through all the sugars and carbohydrates to get into those fat stores and burn them for fuel. Intermittent fasting is an excellent way to jump-start your body into ketosis. Also, periodic intermittent fasting while your body is in ketosis will help it maintain the state because it keeps the carbohydrate levels in the body to a negligible amount. If you're going to start a ketogenic diet, you might want to start it with a 24-

to 48-hour water fast. Drink plenty of water and **consult with your medical doctor or qualified health professional before implementing a ketogenic diet.**

Once your body is in a state of ketosis, you can do intermittent fasting for at least 16 hours per day three to four days per week.

Some people believe you can consume any kind of fat when you're on a keto diet. Nothing can be farther from the truth. Many people load up their plates with bacon and then proclaim, "I'm on keto, so it's healthy." According to Dr. David Friedman in his book *Food Sanity,* if you consume a lot of bacon, you're likely to hear two words that begin with the letter "c" – either "clear" or "cancer." Bacon is NOT a healthy fat. On the other hand, avocado is a healthy fat. An avocado also contains a lot of dietary fiber and other important nutrients to help keep your body healthy.

Dr. David Permutter, M.D., in his book *Grain Brain,* states that the optimal macronutrient ratio will vary from person to person. Some individuals will thrive on a diet with roughly 80 percent of their calories coming from healthy fats and 20 percent from carbohydrates and protein, while others may do better with 60 to 75 percent of their calories coming from fat and the remainder from protein. You'll need to determine which is best for you. Keep in mind that we all have different body chemistries and compositions. What might work for your neighbor might not work for you and vice versa.

Fasting Mimicking Diet

Dr. Valter Longo of the Longevity Institute at the University of Southern California is a leading expert in the study of the "fasting mimicking diet." His research ties together studies in cellular biology with animal studies and human trials to provide an explanation for the numerous benefits of fasting, such as:

- lowering visceral fat
- reducing cancer rates
- improving the immune system
- slowing down the loss of bone mineral density
- increasing longevity

What is Mimic Fasting and How Does It Work?

The fasting mimicking diet follows the same general principles as regular fasting in that you are depriving the body of food in order to take advantage of the health benefits of fasting, like reduced inflammation and fat burning. The primary difference is that instead of eliminating all food for a set period of days or even weeks, you are restricting calories for five days out of the month. This fasting period of five days can be done once a month or practiced every other month to promote health and well-being.

During day one of the diet, calories are restricted to 1,100 calories. For the remaining four days calories are restricted to 800 a day. But it's not only the *amount* of food you eat that is important, but it is also *what* you eat and in what ratios. Different proponents of the diet will recommend different macronutrient ratios. The general recommendation is to eat 1,100 calories that consist of 34 percent carbohydrates, 10 percent protein, and 56 percent fat on day one, and 47 percent carbohydrates, 9 percent protein, and 44 percent fat for the last four days. Others recommend an even higher intake of fat, with as much as 80 percent of calories coming from fat, 10 percent from protein and carbs, respectively. According to Dr. Longo, "The Fasting Mimicking Diet allows the natural process of starvation (autophagy, protection, stem cell regeneration) to occur. You don't interfere with the natural process. That's a key of the Fasting Mimicking Diet."

Are you confused about the Fasting Mimicking Diet? You're not alone. I am too. But here's the good news. Results published in the June 15, 2018, issue of a *Nutrition and Research* article titled, "Effects of 8-hour time-restricted feeding on body weight and metabolic disease risk factors in obese adults: A pilot study," were parallel to those of previous research done on fasting including mimic fasting. The study also found it's easier for you to maintain a 16-hours off, 8-hours on diet compared to other fasting diets, such as the Fasting Mimicking Diet, with the same benefits. This is a huge benefit because many current diets are not sustainable.

David Medansky

One Day (Twenty-Four-Hour) One Meal Intermittent Fasting

Paul and Patricia Bragg recommend a one day (24 hour) fast each week. Here's how it works:

Your 24-hour fast can be from lunch to lunch or dinner to dinner, so long as you abstain from all solid foods. This also means no fruit or vegetable juices. Drink only pure water. Paul and Patricia Bragg recommend that you drink only distilled water. However, because there is some debate about distilled water versus spring water, you can drink spring water if you prefer. My preference is to drink distilled water. This means no flavored enhanced waters or carbonated water.

An exception to drinking only pure water is to add one-third teaspoon of raw honey and one teaspoon of lemon juice. This acts as mucus and toxic dissolver. It is not to help you keep up your strength. It's important to drink copious amounts of water during a fast to flush out the contaminants from your body.

Breaking Your Fast

According to Paul Bragg, at the end of your 24-hour fast, the first food you should eat is a variety of raw vegetables with a base of grated carrots and grated cabbage, because this acts as a broom for cleansing your intestines. It provides the muscles along your gastrointestinal tract something to work with.

Bragg also emphasizes never to break a fast with animal products such as meat, milk, cheese, butter, fish, nuts, or seeds. He recommends raw vegetables such as spinach, kale, chard, or cooked string beans.

You are building a painless, tireless, and ageless body with your 24-hour fast. Patricia Bragg said during an interview that she does her 24-hour fast once a week, on Monday.

To keep your morale high during your 24-hour fast, Paul Bragg, in his book, *The Miracle of Fasting*, recommends you repeat the following affirmations:

- I have this day put my body in the hands of God and Nature. I have turned to the highest power for internal purification and rejuvenation.

218

- Every minute that I am fasting, I am flushing dangerous poisons out of my wonderful body that could do great damage. Every hour that I am fasting, I am happier and happier.
- Hour by hour my body is purifying itself.
- In fasting, I am using the same method for physical, mental, and spiritual purification that the greatest spiritual leaders have used throughout the ages.
- I am in complete control of my body during this fast. No false hunger habit-pangs are going to make me stop fasting. I will carry my fast through to a successful conclusion because I have absolute faith in God and Nature.

Three-Day Fasting

If you're going to do a three-day fast, it should be done under ideal conditions, especially your first long fast. You should be able to rest any time you feel it's necessary and be in a quiet, stress-free environment. During the three days, you should avoid listening to the radio, watching TV, reading, or having company. It's OK to retire to your bedroom and remain in seclusion.

Before your three-day fast, discuss it with your medical doctor or qualified health professional, but don't discuss it with people who aren't qualified to give you advice. You want to avoid letting them project negative thoughts onto you at a time when you need to think positively. Your fasting should be a personal thing.

The most obvious and best-researched benefits of longer fasts are for weight loss: if you're not eating anything, the weight will drop off your body quickly. During the first 24 hours or so, you go through all the glycogen in your liver. After that, your body needs to run on what it has stored, either protein or fat.

For the first few days, weight-loss averages around one to two pounds a day, both because you're shedding water weight and because your body is drawing from your own protein stores for fuel. This is risky because it means breaking down muscles – not only your biceps, but also more essential muscles like your heart. This makes fat by far a preferential energy source, so after a few days, fasting experts say your body turns to its stored fat reserves for energy. Since fat is more energy-dense per pound than protein, weight loss during this phase slows down to a more reasonable but still rapid pace of a little over one pound every two days.

Essentially, a long fast is a way of staying in ketosis for an extended time and forcing your body to rely entirely on its own fat stores instead of dietary fat intake. Being in ketosis makes it easy to lose weight since it suppresses hunger (once you get through the first few days, which are always rough). Fasting also allows you to completely get your mind off food, instead of always thinking about what you're going to eat next and worrying about if you're eating too much.

Long fasting is an effective way to lose a lot of weight quickly, but with a significant caveat: many people proceed to gain it all back again because they just go back to their old obesogenic diet right afterward. Like any other "crash diet," fasting will help you lose weight, but won't help you keep it off unless you also make a long-term change in your diet after the fast is over.

Another benefit of extended fasting is purely mental: for many fasters, it's a way to "re-set" their relationship with food, break free from patterns of emotional eating, or start fresh at the end of the fast. Fasting is part of many religious and spiritual practices because of its value for meditation and mindfulness. Bear in mind that this doesn't happen automatically: it requires a high level of self-awareness and effort on the part of the faster. It's a very useful tool, but it's not a miracle cure.

Still not convinced? Physicians tell people to fast all the time. If you go for a colonoscopy, surgery, or get sick, doctors tell you not to eat for at least 12 to 24 hours before the procedure. Guess what? Nothing bad happens to you because of not eating for a 12- to 24-hour time period.

Resources

If you want more information about how to properly and safely do a three day or longer fast, read Paul Bragg's book *The Miracle of Fasting* and please consult with your medical doctor or a qualified health professional.

The Miracle of Fasting describes the history of fasting, it's benefits, and how to properly fast. If you take nothing else away from this lesson, I'd highly encourage you to obtain a copy and read it. Originally published in 1979, it was the number one health book in Russia for 14 years. Let me repeat that. It was the number one health book sold in Russia for 14 years. It was republished in 2004.

Chapter 14

Putting it All Together

It's not what you say you're going to do that defines you, it's what you do that defines who you are.

Thomas Edison said, "The doctor of the future will give no medicine but will interest his patients in the care of the human frame, in diet and in the cause and prevention of disease." Edison is wrong. The future is now, and we consume more processed foods that are scientifically engineered so that we never are satisfied. These processed foods are deadly.

More than 70 percent of the U.S. adult population is overweight with 41 percent being clinically obese. And it's getting worse. More people are taking medications for preventable diseases and ailments. It's the new normal. I challenge you to be the exception. It's not about my being right or wrong. It's about what you will do – be a part of the new normal or dare to be different.

In previous lessons, you learned what to do and how to reduce weight in a healthy and sustainable manner. In this lesson, you learn how to put it all together. Remember, knowledge without action is worthless. You must use and implement what you have learned about healthy weight loss and how to transform your lifestyle, or this course has been a waste of your time.

This is the story of four people named Everybody, Somebody, Anybody, and Nobody. There was an important job to be done and Everybody was asked to do it. Everybody was sure Somebody would do it. Anybody could have done it, but Nobody did it. Somebody got angry about that because it was Everybody's job. Everybody thought Anybody could do it, but Nobody realized Everybody wouldn't do it. It ended up that Everybody blamed Somebody when Nobody did what Anybody could have done.

What does this have to do with weight loss?

Everything, because Everybody (at least most people) want to lose weight. Anybody who puts forth the time and effort can shed their unwanted pounds. Some of you might blame others such as your spouse, co-workers, boss, or others for your being overweight or obese. Nobody can lose weight for you. You must do this for yourself. You cannot pay Somebody to drink pure water for you, choose healthier whole or holistic foods instead of fast foods or processed foods. Even if Somebody could choose healthier foods for you, they can't chew it for you. In the end, Everybody blames Somebody when Nobody did what Anybody, such as yourself, can do to lose weight in a healthy and sustainable manner.

Here's the simple formula – yes, the one from Dr. David Katz – to attain a healthy weight and maintain it. Do you know it by heart yet?

- Eat holistic (whole) foods,
- Not too much,
- Mostly plants,
- Avoid processed foods,
- Drink lots of pure water, and
- Get adequate sleep.

Simple, yes? But as you've learned, if you attempted to implement it during this course, it's not so easy to do. It's easy to swim with the current, to go with the flow. Today, that means being overweight, or in some cases, obese. It's easy to do what other people do, go where they go, eat what they eat. Especially with the convenience of fast foods and processed foods. But, if you want to successfully reduce weight and keep it off, you've got to swim upstream, against the current, and do what others aren't willing to do. The current is your complacency with your own eating habits. Again, 70 percent of the U.S. adult population is overweight, of which 41 percent are clinically obese. It's an epidemic and it's getting worse. Today, it's the new normal to be fat.

If you don't want to be a part of the new normal, you'll need to go against the flow, because going with the flow is following the herd. Going with the flow is eating fast foods, frozen foods, junk foods, and other addicting processed foods. The flow is taking you downstream to the stagnant waters of poor health, higher risk for a heart attack or stroke, type 2 diabetes, and other ailments that can be prevented and avoided.

Take the path of most resistance. Do what you don't want to do. If you don't want to eat a piece of fruit instead of the candy bar, choose the fruit. Want to eat that delicious fresh baked bread served at the restaurant, choose not to eat it. Don't want to drink more pure water, drink more pure water. Change and improve your daily eating habits until they become new healthier eating habits. Make the healthier choices that you're resisting. No longer let the current, the herd, take you down-stream. Go against your normal tendencies and achieve and maintain a healthy weight. You'll have more energy, feel better, look better, and be able to do more with your kids and grandkids.

As a reminder, these are at least 10 eating behaviors you can change and improve:
- Drink more pure water.
- Avoid processed foods such as deli meats, potato chips, chips of all sorts, cookies, and other snacks.
- Eat more holistic (whole) foods such as fresh (or frozen) vegetables, fruits, and berries. Avoid fruit juices.
- Learn how to read and understand Nutrition Fact labels.
- Reduce your portion sizes. Use a salad plate instead of a dinner plate.
- Eat slower.
- Reduce or avoid alcoholic beverages. Eliminate all sodas from your dietary intake.
- Watch your feelings because they become your thoughts, which become your words. Your words have an impact. They lead to your actions, which lead to your results and eventually to your character.
- Stop eating after 7:00 p.m. or at least three hours before you retire to go to sleep.
- Get adequate sleep.

You can do this! It doesn't matter what I think or what anyone else thinks if you can do it or not. The only person's opinion that matters is yours. Anything is possible. You have choices. I respect your decision.

This is what Jan Miliken wrote to me in December 2018, "I turned 63. I felt old, tired, and depressed, and I had been carrying around some extra weight for a few years. I had given up any hope of taking off those extra pounds. I told myself that I was no longer capable of losing that weight, that I was old and that carrying extra weight was all part of being a senior citizen. But David convinced me otherwise. With his help and support, I have surpassed my goal of a 30-pound weight loss and to date, I have lost 45 pounds without ever feeling deprived or hungry!!! And I no longer feel like a senior citizen either!! Thanks, David, for helping me feel young again."

Your environment does not define you. You've got to put in the effort. You need to immediately turn ideas and inspiration into action and application. Knowledge without action is useless. Have you purchased a self-help product but not put it to use? It becomes shelf help instead of self-help.

There are no excuses or justifications for your being overweight. You are responsible for your weight at all times. You decide what to put into your mouth. If you choose to eat something you know you shouldn't indulge in, it's your emotional immaturity for being irresponsible to properly care for your body. If you travel for business and eat foods you know you should avoid, it's just a B.S. story you tell yourself to justify making poor food choices. Remember the three words to avoid:

Try = You're lying to yourself. You'll either do it or you won't. What matters is doing your best and making more than a "good faith" effort.

Can't = You're already defeated. You've admitted that no matter you do you won't succeed. How do you know if you'll succeed until you make an effort?

But = These are the excuses and justifications you'll use to explain why you failed.

Transformation is never easy. Anyone who tells you otherwise is lying. As you learned, Americans spend $66 Billion on weight-loss products each year ranging from diet pills, to meal plans, to swanky gym memberships. Did you join a gym at the beginning of the year? Almost 80 percent of people who make a New Year's resolution to lose weight or get in better shape fail within the first month.

More than 43 million Americans start a diet or weight-loss program each year. However, 90 to 95 percent of those on diets fail to lose the weight, or if they do, to keep it off.

Diets are a temporary fix to being overweight.

So, while Dr. Katz might have the simple solution to achieving and maintaining a healthy weight, it's not so easy to do. Otherwise, we'd all be thin and healthy.

And by the way, being thin doesn't necessarily mean you're healthy. A thin person can have a drug problem, an eating disorder, be a smoker, or have other health issues. If you want to succeed in achieving a healthy weight and maintaining it, you need to make a lifestyle change.

Earlier in this chapter and in a prior chapter, you learned 10 eating behaviors you can change and improve upon to reduce weight in a healthy manner. You also learned what to do to implement behavior modification. To refresh your memory, the 10 eating behaviors you learned to improve are:

1. Drink more pure water.
2. Avoid processed foods, which includes deli meats, snacks such as pretzels, chips of all kinds, cookies and other quick foods. Avoid the Pop-Tart or donut for breakfast. If you think having a bagel with cream cheese and a glass of orange juice is a healthy breakfast, you'd be wrong. Also, avoid farm-raised fish, beef, and chickens whenever possible.
3. Eat more holistic (whole) foods such as fresh or frozen vegetables, fruits, and berries. Avoid the fruit juices.
4. Learn how to read and understand the Nutrition Fact labels on food products. You might be surprised and shocked to learn what's in the food you're eating, such as aspartame or high-fructose corn syrup.
5. Reduce your portion sizes by using a salad plate instead of a dinner plate. Again, if you put the same amount of

food on the salad plate as the dinner plate, it will appear that there is less food on the dinner plate and more on the salad plate. It's an optical illusion.

6. Eat slower. Put your fork down between each bite. Make a game of seeing how slowly you can eat a meal.
7. Reduce or avoid alcoholic beverages.
8. Watch your feelings because they become your thoughts. Watch your thoughts because they become your words. Watch your words because they make an impact. Your words become your actions which lead to your results. And, your results become your character.
9. Stop eating after 7:00 p.m. or at least three hours before you retire to go to sleep.
10. Get adequate sleep.
11. Avoid microwaved foods whenever possible.

Now you not only know what to do, but how to do it.

Yes, I realize I've repeated this information a few times. Repetition is good because it will re-enforce what you're learning.

Food manufacturers are working against your efforts to reduce weight. Processed foods are scientifically engineered to optimize the amount of salt, sugar, and fat to increase your craving for it. Unfortunately, the human body has evolved to crave foods that deliver just the right amount of saltiness, richness, and sweetness. That's because your brain responds with a reward in the form of endorphins. Howard Moskowitz coined the term "Bliss Point" to refer to this sensation.

Earlier you learned that in 1975 the average supermarket carried about 9,000 food products. Today, the average grocery store sells more than 50,000 food products. The reason there are so many more food products is from the rapid increase in the development of processed foods with grains being chemically engineered. These processed foods are addictive. If you eat mostly processed foods, you become a food junkie. You can never get enough – just like a junkie on heroin. This is the reason you need to eliminate processed foods, or at least reduce the amount you consume, from your dietary intake and increase the amount of whole, unprocessed foods.

The biggest regret people have about losing weight is not starting a year earlier.

The second biggest regret about attaining a healthy weight is not starting now. Ask yourself: if not now, when?

There is never a perfect or right time to begin shedding your unwanted and unhealthy weight. Tomorrow never comes. How many of you have used the excuse or justify delaying your weight loss journey saying, "I'll start on Monday." Or, "I'll start after the holidays?" "After our vacation?" You get the idea. Lemony Snicket said, "If we wait until we're ready, we'll be waiting for the rest of our lives."

Here are the Top 10 excuses people use to delay reducing weight:

1. I'll start after our vacation.
2. I'll start after the holidays.
3. Now's not the right time for me.
4. I'm too busy.
5. I'll start on Monday.
6. It's too expensive or healthy food cost too much.
7. I'll start after our company picnic or party.
8. I'll start after we meet our friends for dinner on Wednesday.
9. Many people who lose weight gain it all back so why bother?
10. I'm always hungry on a diet.

I was fortunate to avoid having a heart attack from being overweight. How many of you know someone who wasn't so lucky?

I was fortunate to avoid having Type 2 diabetes by changing my eating behaviors and reducing weight. Unfortunately, many of my friends and acquaintances weren't so lucky.

Are you pre-diabetic or diabetic? Do you know someone with this condition?

It's estimated that over 29 million Americans have Type 2 diabetes, but 8.1 million may be undiagnosed and unaware of their condition. About 1.4 million new cases of Type 2 diabetes are diagnosed in the United States every year. More than one in every 10 adults who are 20 years or older has Type 2 diabetes. In other words, about 15 percent of the U.S. population are diabetics. What this means is that if you're over age 20 and at a social gathering with 10 other friends, one of you is probably a diabetic.

Here's the rub, many people, maybe even some of you, would rather suffer the consequences of poor health, medical ailments, and even death rather than give up your processed junk food. Research has shown that Oreo cookies are more addicting than cocaine. When they say, "Betcha can't eat just one" referring to potato chips, it's not a dare it's a fact. Can you relate to this?

Now, imagine weighing 24 to 48 pounds less by this time next year. This much I know, you can lose at least two or three pounds per month. So, if you lost just two or three pounds per month for 12 consecutive months, you'd weight 24 to 36 pounds less by this time next year.

The biggest issue many people have along their weight-loss journey is being held accountable. How do you create a culture of being accountable? As suggested earlier, try one or more of these approaches: Ask a friend, relative, co-worker, or another person to be your accountability partner. Or join a group of people who are into modifying and improving their eating behavior to achieve a healthy weight. If you can't find someone to be your accountability partner, or a group to join, start your own group. There are many options available because of Facebook and other social media outlets.

This is how Weight Watchers got started. It was in the early 1960s that Weight Watchers founder Jean Nidetch began inviting friends into her Queens home once a week to discuss how best to lose weight. Today, that group of friends has grown to millions of women and men around the world.

There is a simple solution to holding yourself and others accountable. You can use this process for other areas of your life, such as business or family, in addition to reducing weight. Simple is an acronym that stands for:

S = Set expectations
I = Invite commitment
M = Measure progress

P = Provide feedback
L = Link to consequences
E = Evaluate effectiveness

S = Set Expectations – You and your accountability partner need to understand what is expected of each other. You need to know what is expected so you can be held accountable for those expectations. The more clearly your goals and expectations are defined up front, the less time will be wasted later clarifying, or worse arguing about what is expected.

I = Invite Commitment – Your desire to lose weight doesn't translate into you committing to lose weight. Many people want to lose weight. Few are willing to commit to act or do something about it. If you're not going to commit to reducing weight by modifying and improving your eating habits, no one can hold you accountable. You'll end up making excuses or justifying your poor food choices.

M = Measure Progress – Similar to setting S.M.A.R.T. goals, being held accountable or holding someone accountable needs to have a method to measure performance and progress. Goals are only measurable when they are quantified. You need to be able to measure the results and compare them to the goal to determine if you're succeeding. For example, if you set a goal to shed two pounds each month, and you fail to lose those two pounds, you need to review and see what happened. On the other hand, if you do shed two or more pounds in a month, celebrate all small wins. That does NOT mean going out for a hot fudge sundae or indulging in the food you need to avoid. There are other ways to celebrate such as buying a new outfit or pair of shoes. This was discussed in a prior lesson.

P = Provide Feedback – Feedback won't solve the problem by itself. But a debriefing of the situation will help. To debrief ask yourself these questions:

- What happened?
- How did it make you feel?
- What did you learn from this event or situation?
- How can you use what you learned in the future?

L= Link to Consequences – If you fail to achieve a healthy weight, there will be consequences. The consequences can be in the form of low energy, low self-esteem, higher risk for having a heart attack or stroke, being diagnosed with Type 2 diabetes, contracting some form of cancer, or even death. You can establish other forms of consequences such as paying a fine. As an example, if you fail to lose two pounds in a month you pay $20 to your favorite charity.

E = Evaluate Effectiveness – Review how your process has been handled. Periodically, maybe once a month or every two months, review with your accountability partner what's working and what's not working. Keep what's working and figure out how to correct what's not working. Keep in mind that your weight-loss journey is like running a marathon without a finish line. This is not a diet, which is temporary, this is a lifestyle change through behavior modification.

What obstacle is holding you back from starting your lifestyle transformation?

People who defy the odds have one thing in common. They start. Anywhere, anyhow. They don't care if it's the right time or if the conditions are perfect or if they feel they're being slighted. They start because they understand and recognize that if they can just get some momentum, they can make it work.

Let me tell you a story to illustrate this point. Amelia Earhart, the female aviator from the 1920s, was made what some might consider being an offensive offer one day in 1928. The offer went something like this, "We have someone willing to fund the first female transatlantic flight. Our first choice has backed out. You won't get to fly the plane. You'll be a passenger. We're going to send two men along as chaperones and they'll get paid a lot of money. You won't get paid anything."

Would you have said "Yes" to that offer? That's exactly what Earhart said. She said "Yes."

Amelia Earhart became the first female passenger on a transatlantic flight. The man who made her the offer was George Palmer Putman.

Amelia flew with pilot Wilmer Stultz and mechanic Lou Gordon, from Newfoundland to Wales aboard the trimotor plane "Friendship." Amelia's adventurous attitude and courage were acclaimed around the world. Upon the flight's completion, Amelia wrote the book *20 Hours - 40 Minutes* to tell the story of her experience.

Amelia married George in 1931 but continued to use her maiden name.

Earhart became the first woman to make a solo transatlantic flight in 1932. And, in 1935, she became the first person to fly from Hawaii to the American mainland. By doing so, Amelia became the first person to solo both the Atlantic and Pacific Oceans. Notice I said, "first-person" not "first female." The rest, as they say, is history.

The lesson from this story is that Amelia Earhart said "Yes" to a ridiculous proposal instead of turning her nose at that offensive offer or sitting around feeling sorry for herself.

Are you feeling sorry for being overweight instead of doing something positive to start your lifestyle transformation? Being overweight can be frustrating, even embarrassing. Many of you know what to do to shed your unhealthy and unwanted weight. You might even know how to do it. Yet, you do nothing. What needs to happen to motivate you enough to lose weight?

For me, it was my doctor telling me to lose weight or die. As I mentioned, I succeeded in losing 50 pounds in four months after I failed to lose weight anytime during the prior eight years.

Do you have a million reasons or excuses for not improving your eating habits? Just because starting your transformation isn't exactly to your liking, or you feel you're not ready yet, doesn't mean you get a pass. If you want to create your thinner self and achieve a healthy and sustainable weight, you'll have to start now. Again, you need to ask yourself, if not now, when?

If you're having a tough time losing weight, it is OK to get discouraged. Your body is fighting like heck to keep the weight on. You're being bombarded with TV commercials showing delicious foods at restaurants, fast food joints, and decadent snacks and other goodies.

After all, how often do you see a commercial for fruits and vegetables? Rarely, if ever.

Of course, they'll show you lots of commercial for orange juice. Why? Because as you learned earlier, orange juice is a processed food! It contains natural sugar, but think about this: It takes four to eight medium oranges to make one glass of juice. How many of you would eat four to eight oranges at one sitting? Yet, you'll drink the same amount of sugar and carbohydrates without the fiber in a glass of orange juice and think you're being healthy.

Regardless of all the fancy advertising and marketing for fatting food you need to endure each day, it's not OK to quit. Keep making small adjustments to your daily eating routine, and, if done consistently over a long time, you'll see noticeable results. Henry Ford said it best when he said, "When everything seems to be going against you remember that the airplane takes off against the wind, not with it."

Can we agree you weren't born fat and that you didn't put your excess weight on overnight? Many of you, like myself, put the weight on gradually over several months or years. What makes you think you can get rid of it within a few weeks? If you're believing the hype on TV ads or magazine covers, you're sadly mistaken. Your body is not Amazon Prime. It won't show up in two days.

Walk into any Barnes & Noble or other major bookstore and you'll find hundreds of books about weight loss and dieting. Amazon has more than 50,000 books about health, fitness, and diets. There are hundreds of different diets that claim to work including the following:

- Keto diet
- Paleo diet
- Cabbage soup diet
- South Beach diet
- Mediterranean diet
- Weight Watchers
- Jenny Craig
- Nutrisystem
- Medifast
- Atkins diet
- Zone-Diet
- Vegan Diet

David Medansky

Many people spend a lot of time thinking about which diet is best for them. These same individuals tell themselves that they'll start once they determine which diet they can trust or afford. This is a delay tactic. It is better to focus on results instead of a pretty method.

If your mission is to achieve a healthy weight and maintain it, it doesn't matter how you accomplish it, so long as you do accomplish it. Henry Ford said, "Whether you think you can, or think you can't – your right."

Your mind is the most important part of your body for weight-reduction, but it is the one area most weight-loss programs neglect or ignores. The greatest enemy for reducing weight and shedding those unwanted pounds lives in the grey matter between your ears. This is the primary reason you won't start a weight-loss program. It's because of your mindset. You refuse to believe you can do it. You know what to do, you just refuse to.

To be successful in achieving a sustainable healthy weight you must think in positive terms. Your desire to reduce weight is based on a combination of your thoughts, your feelings, and how those affect your eating habits and actions. This is your mindset.

Do you now view food as fuel for your body? Or, do you still use food for comfort and socializing? Here are some more suggestions for thoughts you can tell yourself:

- I've made the decision to take control of myself – and that includes how I look and how much I weigh.
- I'm committed to achieving a healthy weight by making small adjustments to my daily eating routine until they become new habits.
- I know the first step to achieving a healthy weight is believing I can do it.
- I understand that my words have an impact. Therefore, I will talk positively about myself and avoid negative thinking.
- I begin each day with gratitude.
- I focus on making small adjustments to modify and improve my eating routine.

- I set my weight-loss goals and review them at least once per month.
- I choose to make changes to my unhealthy eating habits and commit to making better food choices.

Is your little voice deep down inside saying, "He's got to be kidding? This won't work for me; this won't last?" That's your negative self-talk. You learned earlier that humans have between 12,000 and 60,000 thoughts per day and that 80 percent of those thoughts are negative.

Imagine, 80 percent of our thoughts are negative or non-supportive. And here I am telling you to reverse that trend because I know you can do it. But it doesn't matter what I think. Because this is what I know: You can change your attitude and change your thought to be supportive and positive so long as you believe it.

Henry Ford said, "There is no man living that cannot do more than he thinks he can." Vince Lombardi said, "Once a man has made a commitment to a way of life, he puts the greatest strength in the world behind him. It's something we call heart power. Once a man has made a commitment, nothing will stop him short of success." Lombardi wasn't talking about football. He was talking about "a way of life." Achieving and maintaining a healthy weight is a way of life.

It's a lifestyle. Remember, once you achieve a healthy weight, maintaining it is a permanent lifestyle. A lifestyle is not a diet. Diets are temporary, extreme, and unsustainable. Your new lifestyle is a break from your past; it's like running a marathon without a finish line. You cannot revert to your old eating habits and retain your newfound health or a healthy body. Because if you do, you'll gain all the weight back, maybe even more just like the other 90 to 95 percent of people who go on diets. You can be in the 5 to 10 percent who succeed.

Stop lying in BED. Bed stands for Blame, Excuses, Denial. As the punchline goes, Denial is not the name of a river in Egypt. Don't be the punchline. Stop lying in BED.

The Standard American Diet (S.A.D.) has left Americans eating too much grain. Grains, such as corn, soy, wheat, rice, bread, pasta, and foods made from these are proven to be a gut irritant causing digestion issues and inflammation. Yet, the U.S. government recommends six to eight servings of grains per day. This is absurd. Even more illogical is that the USDA (United States Department of Agriculture) Food Pyramid Guide, created in 1974, suggested grains comprise the largest portion of our diets. Fortunately, the Food Pyramid Guide was replaced with "MyPlate" in June 2011. MyPlate is the latest nutrition guide from the USDA published by the USDA Center for Nutrition Policy and Promotion.

President Ronald Reagan said, "The nine most terrifying words in the English language are, 'I'm from the government and I'm here to help.'" President Reagan was right. Keep in mind, the Federal Drug Administration (FDA) approves the use of high-fructose corn syrup as an artificial sweetener in food. As the use of high-fructose corn syrup has increased (it's used in just about every processed food product), so have levels of obesity and related health problems. Some wonder if there's a connection.

It is known, however, that too much added sugar of all kinds — not just high-fructose corn syrup — can contribute unwanted calories that are linked to health problems, such as weight gain, Type 2 diabetes, metabolic syndrome, and high triglyceride levels. All of these boost your risk of heart disease.

The Dietary Guidelines for Americans recommend cutting back on added sugar, limiting it to no more than 10 percent of total daily calories. Here's the rub. The daily recommended caloric intake is about 2,000 calories per day for men and about 1,500 calories for women. Yet the average American adult will consume more than 3,600 calories per day.

According to the American Heart Association (AHA), the maximum amount of added sugars you should eat in a day are 150 calories per day or about 37.5 grams for men and 100 calories per day or 25 grams for women.

Starbucks best-selling drink, a Grande (a medium - 16 ounces) Vanilla Latte delivers 250 calories, and 35g of sugar. Another popular drink served by Starbucks is the Java Chip Frappuccino. A Grande Java Chip Frappuccino has 66 grams of sugar nearly double the daily recommended amount.

A Dunkin Donut doughnut will have a minimum of 11 grams of sugar.

Oreos are certainly not the healthiest cookies you could choose. They are made with high-fructose corn syrup, vanillin (fake vanilla) and cheap oils. There are 9 grams of sugar in just ONE (1) Oreo cookie.

Here is a list of 20 popular foods that contain high-fructose corn syrup:

Ready?

- Sodas
- Candy – Snickers has 20 grams of sugar, and M & M's has 18.4 grams in a regular size bag.
- Sweetened Yogurt
- Salad Dressing
- Breads
- Frozen TV dinners, pizzas, and other meals
- Canned fruit
- Juices – As if there isn't enough natural sugar in fruit juice, they add more.
- Boxed dinners such as macaroni and cheese
- Granola bars - Granola consists of rolled oats combined with various other ingredients, such as dried fruit and nuts. Think a granola bar is a healthy snack alternative or meal replacement? Think again. Many companies sweeten them with HFCS.
- Breakfast cereals – When was the last time you checked the ingredients on the Nutrition Fact label? Many cereals are advertised as healthy, but they are often heavily sweetened with HFCS. Some brands contain over 10 grams of sugar in only one serving. It's easy for some people to eat more than the listed serving size, which can put them over their daily sugar limit right at their first meal of the day.
- Store-bought baked goods - Many grocery stores have their own bakery sections with endless donuts, cookies,

and cakes. Unfortunately, HFCS is the sweetener of choice for many store-bought baked goods.
- Sauces and condiments
- Snack foods such as chips, pretzels, cookies, and crackers.
- Cereal bars
- Nutritional bars - Nutrition bars, also known as "energy bars" or "health bars," consist of high-energy ingredients and are meant to be supplemental.
  - They are marketed as meal replacements for individuals who do not have time for a meal but need energy quickly, such as athletes.
  - Unfortunately, HFCS is added to these quite often, which once again stresses the importance of always checking ingredient lists.
- Coffee Creamer
- Energy drinks and sport drinks
- Jam & Jelly
- Ice Cream

What this means for you is you're eating a lot of different foods that all contain high-fructose corn syrup and you don't even realize it.

The average American adult eats more than 3,600 calories per day. Mostly empty, unhealthy calories with little or no nutritional benefits. The recommended daily caloric intake should be 2,000 calories.

Do you look at the calories on a menu at a restaurant before ordering? If you did, you'd be shocked at how many calories you're consuming in one meal. Dr. Bob Martin, during one of his radio shows, said, "If you knew what I knew, you'd do what I do." I'd modify it to be, "If you knew what was in the processed food you consume, you'd avoid it."

When you remove processed foods from your diet and replace them with whole, clean foods, you'll lose weight. You'll be replacing a poor low-performance fuel for your body with better, higher-quality fuel. Think of it as restoring a car or admiring a restored vehicle. Your body is an amazing machine, and given the proper fuel, it can regenerate and restore itself.

You probably provide regular maintenance for your vehicles. Why won't you do the same for your own body? When you start to provide your body with cleaner whole foods instead of fast convenient processed foods here's what you can expect:

- Improved health
- Protection against chronic diseases
- Noticeable weight loss
- Increased energy
- Clearer skin

Would you like to have more energy, feel better and look better? If you do, start watching what you put into your body as fuel. Food is fuel.

After you made the effort to take the time and spend the money for the highest quality food, do NOT use a microwave to cook it. You learned the reasons for avoiding a microwave to heat or cook any food in a previous chapter. The illusion of being too busy is an excuse for you to delay your journey to achieve a healthy and sustainable weight. If not now, when?

Dave Ramsey, a national radio talk-show host and best-selling author about being debt free, likes to say, "If you will live like no one else, later you can live like no one else." Applying Dave's philosophy about money to being overweight: "If you will eat clean whole foods, mostly plant-based, drink pure water, avoid processed foods, and get adequate sleep like other's won't, later you can live an energetic, vibrant, healthy life while others wallow in the stagnant waters of poor health, low energy, low self-esteem, higher risk for a heart attack or stroke, Type 2 diabetes, some forms of cancers, and other ailments that can be prevented and avoided.

Jim Rohn said, "Indecision is the thief of opportunity." Decide now to achieve a healthy weight. Commit to act now. Ask yourself this, "If I delay and put off until tomorrow what I can start today, what might happen?" Here's a hint to your answer. Tomorrow never comes until it's too late.

What does this mean for you? It means if you keep putting off until tomorrow what you should start today, and tomorrow never comes, you'll never start.

What Will Your Weight-Loss Story Be?

A story starts with a hero who wants something. In this story, you are the hero. You want to reduce weight in a healthy and sustainable manner so that you'll have more energy, feel better, look better and improve your overall health. It's been shown that people will always choose a story that helps them survive and thrive. We shall see how your story plays out. What will your life look like if you fail to achieve a healthy weight? What will it look like if you do achieve a healthy weight?

The character in this story, you, has a problem. The problem is being overweight. You've been struggling to solve your problem of being overweight until you meet a guide to help you.

I'm your guide, I am not your hero. My job as your guide is to provide you with a plan, information, and steps to get the job done. Your job of reducing weight.

Every story needs a villain. In your story, the villain is processed foods, fast foods, distractions that cause you to lose your focus and stress. You learned how food manufacturers are scientifically engineering your food to optimize your craving for salt, sugar, and fat and make their products addicting.

I understand your dilemma because I've been where you are. I mastered the skills you must develop to overcome your obstacles and the challenges you'll face to achieve a healthier weight. You have learned about them in this book.

Every person wants to avoid a tragic ending. As your guide, I'm here to help you avoid failure in losing weight. Because if you fail to achieve a healthy weight and maintain it, you end up with Type 2 diabetes, a heart attack or stroke, poor fitting clothes, low energy, and low stamina, embarrassment, even death.

But, if you succeed, you'll likely have more energy and stamina, feel better, be more active, be healthier, maybe happier, and reduce your risk for ailments and illnesses. The choice is yours. The outcome of your weight-loss story will be determined by the choices you make.

Live up to your own expectations, not down to the expectations of others. A Chinese proverb says, "The teacher opens the door, but you have to enter by yourself."

I've opened the door for you to start making small adjustments to your daily eating routines to modify and improve them. It's up to you to walk through the door and act.

You've been given a lot of information to reduce weight in a healthy and sustainable manner. But knowledge without using it is a waste and is worthless. So, go out and implement what you've learned and make it a healthy life.

EPILOGUE

We've Come A Long Way Baby

But We're Heading in the Wrong Direction

According to Dr. David L. Katz, M.D., since the mid-1980s medical research has known that the leading underlying causes of premature death is the overconsumption of *processed food*. Dr. Katz stated, "Diet has been firmly planted on the short list of leading root causes of premature deaths in the United States for the past quarter century. It has evolved to become the number one cause, and around an ever-growing swathe of the world. Imagine actually knowing nothing about the single factor that siphons away the most years from lives, the most life from years in the modern world. If true, it would seem to signal an urgent, desperate need to figure something out fast so that corrective action could be taken."

Yet, long before the Atkins Diet, South Beach Diet, Keto Diet, Paleo Diet, and other modern-day diets, William Banting, a notable English undertaker, proposed weight loss based on a low-carbohydrate diet limiting the consumption of starchy and sugary foods. Notice I said low-carbohydrate diet, not a no-carbohydrate diet. A balanced diet of complex carbohydrates and healthy fats is important.

It was in 1863, more than 150 years ago, that William Banting wrote a booklet called *Letter on Corpulence Addressed to the Public* which contained the plan for the eating habits he followed. Corpulence is defined as a state of being fat or obese. Translated, Banting's book is titled "Letter on Being Fat or Obese Addressed to the Public." *Letter on Corpulence* is perhaps the most influential weight loss book written.

In his booklet, Banting recounted suffering from being overweight and all his failed diets, fasts, spa, and exercise regimens.

He also discussed all his previously unsuccessful attempts that had been based on the advice of various medical experts. He then describes the dietary change which finally worked for him.

Banting undertook his dietary changes at the suggestion of physician Dr. William Harvey. Banting wrote, "My kind and valued medical adviser is not a doctor for obesity, but stands on the pinnacle of fame in the treatment of another malady, which, as he well knows, is frequently induced by the disease of which I am speaking, and most sincerely trust most of my corpulent friends (and there are thousands of corpulent people whom I dare not so rank) may be led into my tramroad." (p24)

His own diet was four meals per day, consisting of meat, greens, fruits, and dry wine. The emphasis was on avoiding sugar, saccharine matter, starch, beer, milk, and butter. Banting reduced his weight from 202 pounds to 156, a total reduction of 46 pounds, based primarily on his daily food intake.

Banting's pamphlet was popular for years to come has been used as a model for modern diets. Banting's booklet, in which he was the very first to outline a low-carbohydrate diet, remains in print as of 2019 and is still available online.

It is hard to believe, but with our increase in knowledge about obesity, nutrition, and exercise, the problems of being overweight and obese are far worse than at any other time in history. This has happened despite mushrooming sales of health club memberships and home gym equipment. There is now a pandemic of increasing weight across the industrialized world.

Americans spend more than $66 billion each year on weight-loss products. Yet, 71 percent of the U.S. adult population (7 out of every 10 adults) and nearly 20 percent (1 out of every 5) school-aged children between 6 and 19 years of age are overweight or obese. This, to me, is not comprehensible nor conceivable given our scientific knowledge of how our bodies function.

The root causes of chronic illnesses that lead to premature death were described by James McGinnis and William Foege in their research paper titled "Actual Causes of Death in the United States" published in *The Journal of the American Medical Association*

(JAMA), December 1993. It was determined by McGinnis and Foege and later substantiated by Ali Mokdad in his article published in 2004, that our poor eating habits and lack of physical activity are the primary causes of premature death and chronic illnesses and diseases.

Here's the kicker, whereas the most recognized and trusted authorities for health and nutrition recommend eating a mostly plant-based diet, and teach how to achieve it, the popular "fad" diets promote eating more meat, butter, cheese, and fat.

So, as the experts bicker among themselves about the "best" diet to follow to reduce weight in a healthy and sustainable manner, I leave you with this thought from Michael Pollan: "Eat food. Not too much. Mostly plants." I'd add: Drink plenty of pure water. If you do this, you'll be just fine. Whatever you decide to do, do it with excellence. Best of health always.

APPENDIX A

Suggestions of Things to Do Besides Eat

- Walk around the block (or parking lot if you're at work)
- Call a friend
- Read a few pages in a book
- Make a list of top 10 reasons to be active
- Take five slow, deep cleansing breaths
- Write in your food journal
- Write down something you did during the week that you're proud of
- Drink a glass or two of pure water
- Chew some gum
- Take a hot shower or hot soothing bath
- Write a letter or email
- Take a nap (unless you're at work lol)
- Recite your Declarations or Affirmations
- Meditate
- Light some candles
- Organize or straighten a closet
- Read some inspirational or motivational quotes
- Play a musical instrument or listen to some uplifting music
- Say a prayer thanking the universe for providing you strength and guidance
- Call your support or accountability partner

APPENDIX B

What's in your food?

Dangerous chemicals, contaminants, and additives are replacing nature's nutrients in the food we eat. The food manufacturers don't see you as a person. They only see you as profit. Dr. David Friedman, author of the number one bestselling book *Food Sanity* said, "The FOOD Industry cares nothing about health and the HEALTH Industry cares nothing about food." I'd add, the only thing both the FOOD and HEALTH industries care about is how to make a profit, your health be damned.

These are some of the cosmetic chemicals used in fast food:

Sodium Stearoyl Lactylate – Found in shampoo and soap. Used in bread dough

Calcium Disodium EDTA – Found in skin products and hair conditioner. Used in fast food sauces, dips and dressings.

Ammonium Glycyrrhizin – Found in facial mask products. Used as a flavor enhancer, flavoring agent, masks bitter flavors and increases the perceived sweetness level of sucrose.

Disodium Phosphate – Found in mascara and mouthwash. Used as a food preservative.

Propylene Glycol – Found in shampoo, mouthwash and hand sanitizer. Provides most of today's foods and beverages their distinctive taste.

Benzoyl Peroxide – Active ingredient in acne creams. Used to bleach wheat flour white. Found in all fast food bread. Recently banned in China.

Beware of Artificial Flavors

Artificial flavors are made in the lab. Artificial flavors come from anything that is inedible, such as petroleum, that is processed to create flavoring chemicals. Food manufacturers prefer to add artificial flavor to their products because a natural flavor almost always costs much more than an artificial flavor. An artificial flavor is comprised of one of the nearly 700 FDA-allowed flavoring chemicals or food additives categorized as "generally recognized as safe," or any of 2,000 other chemicals not directly regulated by FDA but sanctioned for use by an industry group, the Flavor and Extract Manufacturers Association of the United States.

Emulsifiers, solvents, and preservatives used in artificial flavor mixtures are called "incidental additives." This means that the manufacturers do not need to disclose them on food labels. The FDA permits food manufacturers to use synthetic solvents such as propylene glycol. Flavor extracts and food ingredients that have been derived from genetically engineered crops may also be labeled "natural" because the FDA has not fully defined what the term "natural" means.

An emulsifier is a substance that stabilizes an emulsion. It is a food additive used to stabilize processed foods. Emulsifiers made from synthetic sources commonly are added to processed foods such as mayonnaise, ice cream, and baked goods to create a smooth texture, prevent separation and extend shelf life. Some of these emulsifiers are xanthan, Polysorbate 80, lecithin, and carrageenan. If you see any of these ingredients listed on food packaging, avoid eating these foods. For example, polysorbate 80 is listed as an ingredient on ketchup, various ice cream products, chewing gum, gelatin, and other condiments.

Beware of Glyphosate

Glyphosate, the active ingredient in Roundup, is a widely used and harmful herbicide used on crops and other plants to kill weeds. More than 1.4 billion pounds are used on crops each year. Glyphosate residue can be found in your food supply in beef, chicken, pork, farm raised fish, and in packaged foods. Glyphosate gets into animals from the corn and other grains they are fed. It gets concentrated in collagen.

The EPA considers 0.7 parts per million to be safe. However, certain produce, such as corn, soybeans, carrots, and genetically modified organisms (GMOs) have 13.0 parts per million. In other

words, it's extremely toxic to your body. **Do not purchase foods known to have high levels of glyphosate such as:**
- Soy (this means soy products and soy or vegetable oil)
- Corn and corn oil.
- Canola seeds used in canola oil.
- Beets and beet sugar.
- Squash
- Zucchini
- All GMOs

Required Reading
The five books listed below are required reading if you care anything about your health and well-being:
- *Feeding You Lies How to Unravel the Food Industry's Playbook and Reclaim Your Health,* by New York Times best-selling author and founder of FoodBabe.com, Vani Hari
- *Food Sanity How to Eat in A World of Fads and Fiction,* by New York Times best-selling author and host of To Your Good Health Radio, on Radio MD Podcast
- *The Truth About Food Why Pandas Eat Bamboo, and People Get Bamboozled,* by New York Times best-selling author, David L. Katz, M.D., MPH
- *Sugar Blues*, by William Dufty
- *How to Fight Fatflammation!* By Lori Shemek, Ph.D.

APPENDIX C

Motivational Quotes to Keep You Focused

"It is better to offer no excuse than a bad one." George Washington

"A man too busy to take care of his health is like a mechanic too busy to take care of his tools." Spanish Proverb

"If it came from a plant, eat it. If it was made in a plant, don't." Michael Pollan

"Live a good life. And in the end, it's not the years in a life, but it's the life in the years." Abraham Lincoln

"Life isn't about finding yourself. Life is about creating yourself." George Bernard Shaw

"It's not what you say you're going to do that defines you, it's what you do that defines who you are." David Medansky

"Positive action can change every negative situation." Darren Hardy

"Doing your best is more important than being the best." Zig Ziglar

"Success is a choice." Rick Pitino

"One step in the right direction is worth 100 years of thinking about it." T. Harv Eker

"When you improve a little each day, eventually big things occur. When you improve conditioning a little each day, eventually you

have a big improvement in conditioning. Not tomorrow, not the next day, but eventually a big gain is made. Don't look for the big, quick improvement. Seek the small improvement one day at a time. That's the only way it happens - and when it happens, it lasts." John Wooden, Legendary UCLA Basketball Coach

"You make the choice and those choices make you." Darren Hardy

"Be the exception to the overweight epidemic." David Medansky

"Your actions speak so loudly I cannot hear what you are saying." Ralph Waldo Emerson

"I no longer listen to what people say, I just watch what they do." Winston Churchill

"I no longer listen to what people tell me about their diet, I just watch what they eat." David Medansky

"There is nothing more pitiful than a ready and willing mind, but an incapable body." Jim Rohn

"What doesn't get measured, doesn't get done." Darren Hardy

"Don't tell me what you did yesterday or what you'll do tomorrow, show me what you'll do today." David Medansky

"You can't control how you feel. But you can always choose how you act." Mel Robbins

"You can't go back and change the beginning, but you can start where you are and change the ending." C.S. Lewis

"We can't always be perfect, but we can strive to improve each day." David Medansky

"It takes time to create excellence. If it could be done quickly, more people would do it." John Wooden

"Weight is not a behavior. Weight is an outcome." David L. Katz, M.D.

"Whoever wants to reach a distant goal must take small steps." Helmut Schmidt

"A journey of a thousand miles must begin with the first step." Lao Tzu

"Confront the difficult while it is still easy; accomplish the great task by a series of small acts." Tao Te Ching

"Your body only needs food for fuel. So, eat for fuel." Common sense

"Do not let what you cannot do interfere with what you can do." John Wooden

"Compounding is the greatest mathematical discovery of all time." Albert Einstein

"If you keep on doing what you've been doing to lose weight and it's not working, you'll keep on failing so don't be surprised!" David Medansky

"Success comes from knowing that you did your best to become the best that you are capable of becoming." John Wooden

"If you can't pronounce it, you shouldn't be eating it". Michael Pollan

"The true test of a man's [person's] character is what he [they] do when no one is watching." John Wooden

"Small, comfortable, daily steps toward change and improvement in your eating routine and habits will give you weight reduction success." David Medansky

"What shapes our lives are the questions we ask, refuse to ask, or never think to ask." Sam Keen

"Your life comes down to your decisions. If you change your decisions, you'll change your life." Mel Robbins

"If you don't have the time to do it right, when will you have the time to do it over?" John Wooden

"If you can't explain it simply, do it simply, design it simply... it's because you don't understand well enough." Albert Einstein

"What shapes our weight reduction success are the questions we ask, the questions we refuse to ask, and the questions we never think to ask. Often, we don't know what we don't know." David Medansky

"Stay committed to reducing weight and you will succeed achieving a healthy weight and maintaining it." David Medansky

"If you procrastinate when faced with a big difficult problem...break the problem into parts and handle the one part at a time." Robert Collier

"Intention is the first step to reducing weight. Commitment is the second step. The third step is action. Celebrate achieving small weight reduction goals is the fourth step. Follow through is the fifth step." David Medansky

"Nothing will work unless you do." John Wooden

"It is also important to remember that "yo-yo diets" that lead to rapid weight loss fluctuation are associated with increased

mortality. Instead of engaging in the next popular diet that would last only a few weeks to months (for most people that includes a ketogenic diet), try to embrace change that is sustainable over the long term. A balanced, unprocessed diet, rich in very colorful fruits and vegetables, lean meats, fish, whole grains, nuts, seeds, olive oil, and lots of water seems to have the best evidence for a long, healthier, vibrant life." Marcelo Marcus, M.D., Harvard Health Blog, *Ketogenic diet: Is the ultimate low-carb diet good for you?* posted July 27, 2017, updated July 6, 2018

"It's what we learn after we know it al... That really counts." John Wooden

"People often say that motivation doesn't last. Well, neither does bathing - that's why we recommend it daily." Zig Ziglar

"If you want to be thinner, don't listen to overweight people." David Medansky

"For every promise, there is a price to pay. If you want the promise, be willing and eager to pay the price." Jim Rohn

"Failure is not fatal, but failure to change might be." John Wooden

"For things to improve, you have to improve. For things to change, you have to change. For things to get better, you have to get better." Jim Rohn

"Self-discipline is the ability to make yourself do what you should do when you should do it, whether you feel like it or not." Elbert Hubbard, Editor, Publisher, and Founder of Roycroft Arts and Crafts Community

"If you wear out your body where are you going to live?" Dr. Bob Martin, Certified Clinical Nutritionist (C.C.N.), host of "The Dr.

Bob Martin Show", the largest syndicated alternative health show in the U.S.

"Do what you HATE to do but do it like you LOVE it." Mike Tyson
"Most people's dreams die of fear not failure." Robert W. Jones, Network Together Founder

"Procrastination is a silent killer." Traci Bogan

APPENDIX D

I Begin the Day...

Read the words below, out loud, to start each new day.

- I begin the day expecting amazing things.
- I begin the day being grateful for what I have and what I will receive.
- I begin the day open to receiving new ideas, new information, and new connections.
- I begin the day letting go of what's not serving me, some refer to this as "bless & release."
- I begin the day being a positive influence on others.
- "I am whole, perfect, strong, powerful, loving, harmonious, [grateful, healthy] and happy." Charles Haanel
- Napoleon Hill began his day reciting, "O Divine Providence, I ask not for more riches, but more wisdom with which to make wiser use of the riches you gave me at birth, consisting in the power to control and direct my own mind to whatever ends I desire."

APPENDIX E

Food Journal

Date: _____   Morning weight: _____

Day of week: _____

Juice of one lemon Optional _____   Tbsp. Apple Cider Vinegar Optional _____   Drink eight 8 oz. glasses of Water! ⊔⊔⊔⊔⊔⊔⊔⊔

Breakfast	What time did you eat? _____
What did you eat?	Protein: _____ Vegetable(s): _____ Starch: _____
How much did you eat?	Protein: ____ Oz. Vegetable(s): _____ Cup Starch: _____ Pieces/Cups: _____
Where did you eat?	Kitchen Table: __ Couch: __ Car: __ Restaurant: __ Other: _____
What were you doing?	Just Eating: __ Texting: __ Driving: __ Watching TV: __ Other: _____
Describe your mood.	Stressed __ Anxious: __ Excited: __ Happy: __ Sad: __ Other: _____
Snack – Mid-Morning	Almonds/Nuts _____ Fruit: _____ Cheese _____ Other: _____
Lunch	What time did you eat? _____
What did you eat?	Protein: _____ Vegetable(s): _____ Starch: _____
How much did you eat?	Protein: ____ Oz. Vegetable(s): _____ Cup Starch: _____ Pieces/Cups: _____
Where did you eat?	Kitchen Table: __ Couch: __ Car: __ Restaurant: __ Other: _____
What were you doing?	Just Eating: __ Texting: __ Driving: __ Watching TV: __ Other: _____
Describe your mood.	Stressed __ Anxious: __ Excited: __ Happy: __ Sad: __ Other: _____
Snack – Mid-Afternoon	Almonds/Nuts _____ Fruit: _____ Cheese _____ Other: _____
Dinner	What time did you eat? _____
What did you eat?	Protein: _____ Vegetable(s): _____ Starch: _____
How much did you eat?	Protein: ____ Oz. Vegetable(s): _____ Cup Starch: _____ Pieces/Cups: _____
Where did you eat?	Kitchen Table: __ Couch: __ Car: __ Restaurant: __ Other: _____
What were you doing?	Just Eating: __ Texting: __ Driving: __ Watching TV: __ Other: _____
Describe your mood.	Stressed __ Anxious: __ Excited: __ Happy: __ Sad: __ Other: _____
Snack – After Dinner	Fruit _____ Berries: _____ Yogurt: _____ Other: _____

Day in Review: _____
_____

About the Author

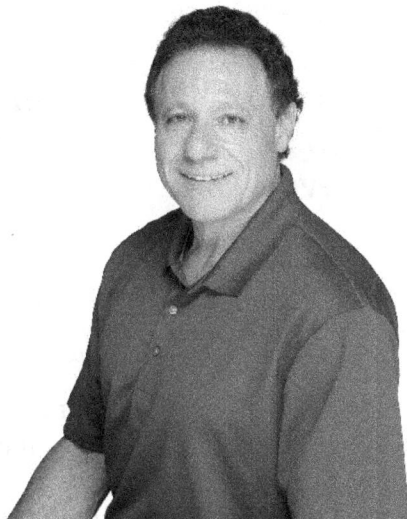

In July 2016, David Medansky, a retired divorce attorney, weighed 217 pounds. His doctor told him to lose weight or find another physician because he didn't want David dying of a heart attack on his watch. Within four months, Medansky dropped 50 pounds. Being an international best-selling author, he wrote about his inspirational weight-reduction journey in his book, *Discover Your Thinner Self*. His new book, *If Not Now, When?* sets forth scientifically proven, common sense, every day, practical principles that will make a significant impact on your weight reduction journey.

Born and raised in the Chicago metropolitan area, Medansky now helps others achieve their weight reduction success. For more information, visit www.CreateYourThinnerSelf.com.

He resides in the Phoenix metropolitan area with his wife.

The key to your weight reduction success is your Encore – It's what you do after you shed the pounds to keep them off.

David Medansky

In Memoriam

*"Some people come into our lives and quickly go.
Some people stay for a while and move our souls to
dance. They awaken us to a new understanding,
leave footprints on our hearts, and we are never,
ever the same."*

Flavia Weedn

Kevin K. Allen, Founder and President/CEO of
Listen University

Kevin Allen lost his battle with cancer in May of 2019.
Kevin made a major impact on thousands of lives,
including mine. The Universe was smiling favorably upon me the
day I was introduced to Kevin, and I will never be the same.
Without my good fortune to meet Kevin, this book would not have
been written. Kevin and the partners at Listen University were
gracious to offer me an opportunity to create a course about healthy
and sustainable weight reduction for Listen University's program.
Those lessons are the foundation and inspiration for the material
presented in this book. Thank you, Kevin, for your generosity,
inspiration, and support.

Acknowledgments

I am grateful and blessed that **Dr. David Friedman**, B.S., N.D., D.C., author of the international award-winning, number one bestselling book, *Food Sanity,* and host of *To Your Good Health Radio* on Radio MD Podcast, has taken the time to communicate with me about what's really going on in the food industry. Dr. Friedman awakened me to a new understanding about eating healthy. He's been an inspiration for me to help others achieve a healthy lifestyle. I appreciate Dr. Friedman's words of encouragement to move forward with this book and make an impact on the lives of others.

What Now?

Don't Let This Book Become Shelf Help.

The Medansky Approach for Reducing Weight – Back to Basics

I hoped you enjoyed reading this book. More importantly, I am optimistic you will implement the lessons into your daily eating routine to achieve a healthier weight. It is my experience, however, that reading alone will not make the difference you are looking for to achieve your weight reduction goal. Reading this book, or other books is a start. If you want to succeed in shedding your extra pounds, it's your actions that matter. Ralph Waldo Emerson said, "Your actions speak so loudly I cannot hear what you are saying."

The hardest part of a thousand-mile journey is starting. Newton's First Law of Motion states in part that an object will remain at rest unless acted upon by an external force. It's a statement about inertia, that objects will remain in their state of motion unless a force acts to change the motion. Most people fail to reduce weight and improve their lifestyle because it's hard to get started. Napoleon Hill once asked an audience what is the average number of times a person will attempt to achieve a new goal? After several members of the audience gave wrong answers, he told them the answer is less than one. You see, even though most people want to improve their lives, reduce weight, and accomplish more, they tell themselves they can't and never make an attempt by starting.

The next challenge most people encounter is staying on track with their weight reduction journey. Newton's Second Law of Motion states that a body will remain in motion unless acted upon by an outside force. For too many folks, there are many outside forces detracting from them staying focused such as family obligations, work-related issues, holidays, special events like weddings, anniversaries, and birthdays as well as other detrimental influences.

Mark Twain said, "Twenty years from now you will be more disappointed by the things you didn't do than by the ones you did do." If you apply Mark Twain's wisdom to eating healthier, you will be more disappointed that you didn't eat healthier and put the proper fuel in your body 20 years from now than if you start today. We all believe we are infallible or invincible until we are confronted with a debilitating illness, lack mental clarity, experience low energy, or are tired of being sick and tired. My wish for you is that you enjoy excellent health throughout your entire life.

Throughout this book, you learned 10 eating behaviors you can modify to improve your eating habits and make healthier choices. You learned that according to Dr. David Katz, M.D., who refers to Michael Pollan, a simple solution to reduce weight in a healthy and sustainable manner is to:

- Eat holistic food
- Not too much
- Mostly plant
- Avoid processed foods and
- Drink lots of pure water

Simple yes? But, as you probably discovered, not so easy to do.

You learned how to read Nutrition Fact labels and how the food manufacturers are scientifically engineering processed food to optimize people's cravings for sugar, salt, unhealthy fat, and texture. You also learned how water may contribute to your inability to reduce weight.

Thank you for spending your valuable time reading this book. I wish you enormous success along your weight reduction journey and superb health. Based on my experience, what I've learned is that most people left on their own tend *not* to accept or make change very well. Much like athletes, we all need a coach or coaches to improve. Michael Jordan had a coach when he played basketball. Serena Williams has a coach to help her improve her tennis game. Tiger Woods has a coach. Those who succeed in reducing weight and keeping it off have a coach or accountability partner. It's extremely difficult to do it alone. That's why I am making myself available to be your coach and/or accountability partner.

According to Darren Hardy, only five percent of people ever seek out and invest in materials or programs to improve themselves. Fewer will read a book cover to cover or finish a program. The statistics prove that you are atypical because you have read this book.

If you're ready to make the commitment to have a greater impact on your weight reduction journey, transform your life, and avoid this book becoming shelf help, read on.

You see, the best way I can make a difference for people committed to shedding their extra weight is to help people make lifestyle changes to their eating habits by keeping them accountable, providing support, keeping them focused and on track, and giving information. So, I've designed a program for you to become one of my success stories.

I have helped countless numbers of people reduce weight in a healthy and sustainable manner without needing to order special foods or products, follow an exercise program, count calories, or do food exchanges. I've been where you're at when it comes to shedding weight. I understand the accountability and support you need to succeed in reducing weight with less stress and irritability. I also know what mindset challenges you will be facing at each stage of your weight reduction journey, such as the dreaded weight plateau. Or, what happens if you drift from your healthy eating habits and cheat. I've designed my program to help you overcome these obstacles with confidence. I'm looking forward to helping you succeed.

With my program, you will get weekly private, personal, and confidential telephone calls to keep you accountable, provide support, and give you information about making healthy food and beverage choices. You'll also get access to step-by-step lessons that you can review at your convenience to keep you focused shedding those extra pounds.

When you enroll in this program, make the commitment to improve, and change your daily eating habits, you'll get results. I'll teach you how? This program is different than diets which are temporary, extreme, and unsustainable. Our approach is realistic, attainable, and sustainable. Once you get rid of those pounds, you might consider reviewing your wardrobe and update it with some new choices, reflecting how good you feel with your weight reduction, or get a makeover.

With this VIP Program, I will create a weekly menu, recipes, and shopping list individualized for you based on your personal likes and dislikes. In addition to weekly private, personal, and confidential telephone calls, you will get two quotes each week to help you stay focused and motivated.

I've helped individuals transform their figure and health. If you're ready to invest in yourself, to find out more and to secure your spot, please send me an email at davidmedansky@gmail.com or call David at (602) 721-5218.

Referrals are the core of my business,
please don't keep me a secret.

Who do you know that might benefit from this program?

No Risk Guarantee: Your first month is **FREE** when you enroll and use the redeem code 1FMCYTS upon checkout. Enroll at: https://createyourthinnerself.com/weight-reduction-program.

Please join our weight reduction community to get more tips, ideas, and information about shedding your extra pounds at my Facebook page, https://www.facebook.com/thinnerself/.

www.ingramcontent.com/pod-product-compliance
Lightning Source LLC
Chambersburg PA
CBHW060314030426
42336CB00011B/1043

9 781733 738859